Contents

Illustrations

Figures

Table

Note on Yoga Terms and Translations

The reader will encounter many Sanskrit words related to yoga terms and concepts in this book. In keeping with a common practice in many English print and online publications about yoga (other than those by trained yoga scholars), I simply anglicize the Sanskrit words without diacritical marks. Instead, I indicate the Sanskrit words in italics, followed by the English translation upon their first appearance in parentheses, such as *savasana* (Corpse Pose). Exceptions to this approach include capitalizing Sanskrit terms in Roman type when used as proper nouns, such as Hatha Yoga, as well as terms that have made their way into common usage, like the word "yoga" itself. Unless otherwise noted, I have used B. K. S. Iyengar's translations of yoga words, terms, and concepts.

Acknowledgments

So many people helped me bring this book to press that I hesitate to even begin naming them. Still, since the project could have only come to fruition with the support of people who maintain archives and special collections, my first round of thanks goes to those who preserve such historic documents in physical spaces. They make it possible for a researcher like me to study and actually touch history. On my first visit to the Foyle Menuhin Archive at the Royal Academy of Music in London during a spring break trip to London in March 2015, I discovered a box simply marked "yoga" full of uncatalogued photos and letters that revealed a close student-guru relationship between Yehudi Menuhin and B. K. S. Iyengar. I am especially grateful to two dedicated archivists in London, Andrew Neilsen and Ian Brearey, who lent expert and steadfast support as I sifted through all the material there. On another research trip to the Ramamani Iyengar Memorial Yoga Institute (RIMYI) in Pune, India, in January 2018, Prashant Iyengar and Abhijata Iyengar (B. K. S Iyengar's son and granddaughter, respectively) kindly gave me access to the binder containing letters from Menuhin to Iyengar. Without support from these archivists and collectors on both sides of the world, London and Pune, I would never have been able to piece together this story.

My next round of thanks goes to the yoga teachers and mentors who directly and indirectly guided my work. Kathleen Pringle first scouted out the Menuhin letters at RIMYI in 2016. Two years later, after I was able to travel to Pune myself to study Menuhin's letters, Steve Jacobson helped me overcome communication challenges to secure authorization from Prashant to reproduce some of these documents by hand-delivering a letter. When the book was already in production, Lois Steinberg helped expedite permission from the Iyengars for three additional images I had discovered after my trip to India. Kquvien DeWeese read an early draft of the "Yoga Primer," and Anna Leo read an early draft of the chapter on the soul connection between Menuhin and Iyengar. Nancy Mau spent time in her yoga classes tracing Iyengar's lineage to his guru Krishnamacharya. These yoga teachers, along with many others, helped me to think about and frame this book in the context of my own yoga practice.

I am extremely thankful to people at Emory University for supporting my research for this book: Michael Elliott, past dean of Emory College of Arts and Sciences, helped to secure major funding from the Mellon Foundation to support research in the humanities and approved my Winship Award in fall 2022 to complete the manuscript; Sarah McKee, past senior associate director of publishing at the Fox Center for the Humanistic Inquiry, provided unwavering direction with the Manifold edition of the book as well as ongoing editorial help; Mae Velloso-Lyons, who most recently stepped into that position, helped prepare the final print images; Allison Adams provided assistance through targeted grants and workshops aimed at supporting faculty projects in her role as director of research and scholarly writing in Emory's Center for Faculty Development and Excellence; Yang Li at the Emory Center for Digital Scholarship created the digital version of this book, and Steve Bransford filmed the violin videos in chapter 4; Catherine MacGregor, my undergraduate student research assistant, demonstrated Menuhin's instructions in those videos and enthusiastically accompanied me on a trip to the Menuhin Archive; and Stephen Crist, chair of the Department of Music, made the initial suggestion I visit the Menuhin Archive in London in 2015, encouraged my ongoing research, and ensured annual faculty research travel grants.

Many thanks to SUNY Press, especially Richard Carlin, for supporting this project and partnering with us at Emory on the digital version of the book. I am also grateful to Lesley McAllister and Suzanne Newcombe for the time and care they gave to read the final manuscript; through their yoga expertise, they directed invaluable comments and suggestions to strengthen and clarify many points.

Finally, I am deeply grateful to my family members who have supported me throughout every stage of this project: my sister Karen Wendland Dix, who was with me on that initial London trip in 2015, read early drafts of the manuscript, and, along with my brother-in-law Vince Dix, offered invaluable feedback about tone for my target reader; my brother Don Wendland, who patiently listened to initial ideas about "my man Yehudi" and critiqued second drafts of chapters; my sister Heidi Lee

Burroughs and brother-in-law Don Burroughs, who are always a source of love and spiritual inspiration to me; and my husband Pat Webster, who the Higher Power brought into my life the same year I started this project and has stood by me through all its ups and downs.

Introduction

Yehudi Menuhin and Yoga

In 2001, when I first began to get serious about practicing yoga, I bought B. K. S. Iyengar's book *Light on Yoga* at the Iyengar yoga studio where I had been taking classes in Atlanta. In 1966, B. K. S. Iyengar was one of the modern world's most important yoga gurus, and he had written a guide for aspiring yoga practitioners, complete with 602 illustrative photos, succinct instructions, and commentary on yoga philosophy. I wanted to dig in and study for myself what the great guru had written. As I dutifully opened the book to the front matter, I gasped in surprise at the heading, "Foreword by Yehudi Menuhin." Wait, Yehudi Menuhin? The world-famous child prodigy and concert violinist? I still had some old LP recordings of his from the 1970s. What did Menuhin have to do with yoga, and why did he write the foreword to this book, considered by many to be the Bible of yoga? I eagerly read on.

It turns out that the great violinist had been practicing yoga and studying with Iyengar for fifteen years by the time he wrote that foreword. I would later find out that Menuhin, in addition to being one of the most famous musical geniuses of the twentieth century, was also one of the earliest and most influential practitioners of yoga in Europe. Menuhin had first discovered yoga in 1952, before it was widely practiced in Europe or the United States, and he was instrumental in bringing yoga and the work of B. K. S. Iyengar to the West. His brief two-page foreword, which includes a discussion of Menuhin's own connection to yoga, gave me insight not only into the practice as taught by Iyengar but also into the practice of one of the world's greatest musicians, something that spoke to me strongly as a musician myself.

And so, curious to learn more about Menuhin's engagement with yoga, I decided to explore more fully the connection between the two seemingly disparate disciplines of music and yoga through the lens of Menuhin's life and work. I began to investigate how and why Menuhin came to yoga and the deep teacher-student relationship he developed with Iyengar. I read Menuhin's published writing, and I studied his unpublished letters and essays housed in archives at the Royal Academy of Music in London and at the Iyengar Institute in Pune, India. I began to understand how forward looking Menuhin was in the way he bridged Eastern and Western thought and by the way he put such thought into musical action. As both a great musician and a benevolent spirit, he became a kind of role model for me as I endeavored to take my own yoga practice into my life and work.

Who Is Yehudi Menuhin?

Born in 1916, Yehudi Menuhin's name may only vaguely resonate today with people born after 1970. As one of the world's most famous twentieth-century child prodigies, however, Menuhin was a household name in the United States and Europe in the 1920s and 1930s. Following his public debut in 1924 in San Francisco, the child prodigy established an international concert career at major halls in New York, Paris, and Berlin. His stellar concert career continued into his adolescent and early adult years as he performed around the world in the United States, Europe, Australia, New Zealand, South Africa, and Latin America.

Unlike many other child prodigies, Menuhin's musical career continued into his adult years and for his entire life right up to his death in 1999. His strong presence as a performing violinist and conductor, a festival organizer, and a teacher impacted the musical world. He continuously maintained an international concert career, playing for audiences at major concert halls, heads of state, and royalty. He even conducted once for the Pope. Numerous biographies and documentary films recount Menuhin's life and work, and in 1996 he published the autobiography *Unfinished Journey: Twenty Years Later* to update his first edition. Most recently the multi-language companion book *Passion Menuhin: The Album of a Life* (2016) accompanies an astounding compilation of Menuhin's landmark recordings and films from 1929 to 1998 in honor of his centennial.[1]

Beyond his musical genius, Menuhin possessed an insatiably curious mind. He pondered, lectured, and wrote about a broad array of issues concerning politics, education, and the environment. As a great citizen of the world, he championed many humanitarian causes and zealously worked to promote peace and unity around the globe. He was a visionary and a humanist committed to reaching the public through his music, writing, and teaching, and he believed music had the power to transform people's lives and provide spiritual healing to a broken world. Throughout his life he was awarded many honors to recognize his great contributions, including twenty honorary doctorates from such prestigious institutions as Oxford University, Cambridge University, and the University of St. Andrews. In his adopted country of the UK, Queen Elizabeth II made him an honorary Knight of the British Empire in 1965; he was knighted Sir Yehudi in 1985 and received the Order of Merit in 1987; and he was inducted into the House of Lords as Lord Menuhin of Stoke d'Abernon in 1993. Menuhin was a passionate promoter of music and education, and his legacy lives on today. The Gstaad Menuhin Festival & Academy remains an important standing international music festival. The Yehudi Menuhin School in England, which he founded in 1963, continues to provide a superbly holistic musical education for young people, while the Yehudi Menuhin International Competition for Young Violinists offers one of the most prestigious music prizes in the world.

I first heard about Menuhin in the 1970s when I was an undergraduate music student. I listened to his classical recordings, along with the other great violinists of his era like David Oistrakh, and I heard about his pioneering "world music" record *West Meets East* (1966) with sitarist Ravi Shankar. Although I continued to come across Menuhin in my work as a musician and academic, it was not until I encountered his name in Iyengar's *Light on Yoga* that I began to investigate his life and work in detail. This book is a result of my research into the connection between Menuhin's life as a brilliant musician and as a dedicated yoga practitioner. While Menuhin's musical life and work from his early years as a child prodigy to his adult years as a performer, educator, and humanitarian have been written about, the link between his life, his music, and his yoga practice is wholly unexamined.

Before I started to practice it myself, I thought yoga was for lightweights—people who were not really serious about physical exercise or only did it for stretching. Although a musician and college professor by training, I have also been very athletic for most of my life. By my early thirties, I was an avid runner, swimmer, and cyclist. I cross-trained. I competed in road races and triathlons. I ran two marathons. But in my early forties, things started to change. I didn't slow down much, but my body did begin to tighten even as my mental awareness deepened. As I approached middle age, I experienced a shift in my perspective about what is really important in life, which often takes root for people around this time, and as my body stiffened, I began to reconsider my earlier judgments about yoga. At age forty-three, I decided to give yoga a chance, and it didn't take long to see that my earlier perspective on it was wrong (like many more things to come). I soon learned that yoga is a physically challenging discipline and is about much more than stretching. I learned that yoga is ultimately about quieting the mind into a state of awareness of the timeless moment. Yoga philosophy turned out to resonate with my own belief system, and I went on to study yoga as a spiritual practice. Today, after practicing yoga for over twenty years, I can say that it has profoundly changed my life physically, mentally, and spiritually.

Scope of the Book

I hope this book will appeal to a wide audience of readers who are drawn to music, yoga, and the intersection between the two topics. It provides music researchers and students with a fresh view of Menuhin's life and work through the lens of his yoga practice, supported by archival evidence from Menuhin's photos, letters, and lectures and by the violinist's autobiographical and pedagogical books and articles. *The Power of Practice* also offers yoga practitioners an inside view of B. K. S. Iyengar, one of the most renowned yoga gurus of the past century, through his teacher-student relationship with Menuhin, again documented by my archival research. For spiritual seekers in general, I hope the book delivers a good read about the two prominent figures in the story, Menuhin and Iyengar, and a compelling story about how the practice and philosophy of yoga may apply to everyday life in general.

I wrote this book because I thought others might need a champion like Menuhin in their lives, especially in our politically polarized and spiritually fragmented world. For millions of yoga practitioners around the world, Menuhin's example reaches beyond just an individual's personal quest for well-being and taps into a greater societal movement of people pursuing new approaches to physical and spiritual health in their lives. In many yoga studios, teachers weave in statements like "find your own way to apply yoga to life" as they give instructions to "straighten your legs" or "observe your breath." Finding helpful examples of what this kind of integration can mean for a Westerner is often difficult.[2] Yehudi Menuhin, however, represents a notable example of someone who embodied many yogic principles in his life and work beginning in the early 1950s, when yoga was hardly known in the West. He sought out ways to integrate yoga not only into his personal approach to well-being but also into his influential work as a musician. In this book, I hold up Menuhin as a relevant case study to show how people can draw on such connections for their own paths of holistic well-being.

I have tried to write this book in accessible language and to avoid deep technical material about both yoga and music, although many yoga terms and concepts are sprinkled through the chapters in Sanskrit with English translations. Chapter 1 of the book, "Soul Connection: Menuhin's Yoga Practice with B. K. S. Iyengar," introduces the reader to the lifelong relationship and connection between Menuhin and Iyengar, from the impact of their initial meeting in 1952 until Menuhin's death in 1999. Chapter 2, "Early Influences and Career: Menuhin's Path to Embracing Yoga," recounts Menuhin's early years with an eye toward what factors may have drawn him to yoga in the first place. Chapters 3, 4, and 5 delve into how Menuhin integrated his musical and yogic disciplines in the dimensions of body, mind, and spirit, respectively, as I analyze and interpret Menuhin's life and work through the lens of the three paths of yoga—*karmayoga* (Yoga of Action), *jñanayoga* (Yoga of Knowledge), and *bhaktiyoga* (Yoga of Devotion)—as thematic frames that align with Menuhin's roles as a performing musician, an educator, and a spiritual believer. Chapter 3, "Yoga Path of Action: Menuhin's Musical Performances," looks at how Menuhin integrated yoga into his actions and accomplishments as a performer of classical music, organizer of music festivals, promoter of world music, and advocate for his guru. Chapter 4, "Yoga Path of Knowledge: Menuhin's Teachings and Writings," recounts how Menuhin applied the knowledge he gained through his yoga practice and study to forge a unique educational mission, including the Yehudi Menuhin School and two books on violin playing. Chapter 5, "Yoga Path of Devotion: Menuhin's Philosophical and Spiritual Beliefs," explores how Menuhin's belief system integrated many yogic concepts of devotion, as reflected through his great humanitarian work and his own writings and lectures.

Finally, a word of explanation about the word "practice" in the title of this book. Anyone who excels on a musical instrument, in a competitive sport, or with any kind of challenging physical discipline knows practice is the key to mastery. But in my use of the term "practice" here I go beyond the meaning of the physical repetition needed for training the body. I use the word to describe how one applies mental disciplines and spiritual principles in their life and actions to embrace a holistic body/mind/spirit meaning. As the power of practice in Menuhin's two disciplines of music and yoga transformed his life and work, I hope his story will inspire readers to find spiritual intersections in their own lives and work that will empower them to make our world a better place.

Chapter 1

Soul Connection

Menuhin's Yoga Practice with B. K. S. Iyengar

Yehudi Menuhin (1916–1999) and B. K. S. Iyengar (1918–2014) established a soul connection when they first met on March 5, 1952. The historic meeting took place in the capital city of the Indian state of Maharashtra, then named Bombay,[1] through the connections of mutual friends and at the request of Menuhin. Upon an invitation from Indian prime minister Pandit Jawaharlal Nehru, Menuhin was on tour in India for the Famine Relief Fund, and, since he had already developed an interest in yoga, was eager to "meet an expert."[2] Iyengar traveled ten hours from his home in the town of Pune to meet Menuhin in Bombay. The violinist should have known immediately that he had met his match with the yoga guru, as he writes how when Iyengar "appeared in my rooms one morning and straight away made it clear, with a kind of rustic authority, that the 'audition' to follow was mine as much as his."[3]

Iyengar, in fact, had never heard of Menuhin. So, for all of the violinist's fame, to Iyengar he was just "another Western body knotted through and through."[4] Menuhin had planned to give Iyengar only five minutes out of his busy schedule, so the guru simply had him lie down and put him in *savasana* (Corpse Pose). Menuhin recounts: "One hour later I awoke, feeling more refreshed than I had felt for ages. Like the other pedagogical 'recognitions' of my life, this one too began with the casting of a kind of spell."[5] Upon Menuhin's request, Iyengar returned the next day, and so began the lessons and a lifelong relationship.

Through Menuhin's connection to Iyengar, yoga would come to play a critical role in the violinist's understanding of his body and his body's relationship to his music. As Menuhin himself makes clear in his writings, his discovery of yoga at the age of thirty-six had a fundamental impact on him, and he eagerly embraced the discipline to establish a regular, ongoing practice that he diligently maintained for the rest of his life. But Menuhin's engagement with yoga penetrated more deeply beyond the body as he channeled his yoga practice into many of his life experiences, questions, and struggles. Beyond his physical practice, Menuhin also absorbed and embodied deeper yogic principles exemplified in his musical life and work. As an immensely important public figure with global renown, his advocacy for diversity and cultural exchange, along with his promotion of yoga itself in Europe and the United States, extended his influence as a powerful force for good far beyond the concert stage and into the realms of spiritual practice, philosophical thought, and social justice. Indeed, as Chapter 5 discusses in detail, many yogic principles form central cornerstones of the philosophy and spiritual devotion Menuhin expresses in his papers, letters, and lectures, such as how a musical artist may channel the Divine Spirit to affect a transcendental experience in a listener.

A Yoga Primer

It is an understatement to say that yoga has become a mainstream and popular form of fitness. Still, the word "yoga" is something of a catchall for a number of different practices today. Print and online yoga publications abound, along with thousands of YouTube instructional videos. The commercial market is flooded with special yoga products like clothes, gear, music, and tours. The United Nations has even declared June 21 (appropriately the summer solstice) the International Day of Yoga.[6] A 2017 study claims that in the US alone more than twenty million people practice yoga, seeking greater flexibility, general conditioning, stress relief, improved overall health, and physical fitness.[7] The Broadway singer-actress Kelli O'Hara testifies about how she practices yoga before going onstage,[8] and many world-famous celebrities are known to practice yoga, including Sting, Tom Hanks, Madonna, Justin Timberlake, Lady Gaga, and Beyoncé.[9]

Today, people practice a huge variety of yoga types, both in India and around the world. Even a simple internet search on "types of yoga" yields bewildering results, and sources disagree on how many types there actually are (some references put the number at as few as six, while others note as many as eleven). The most common yoga names people hear include Ashtanga Yoga, Bikram ("hot") Yoga, Hatha Yoga, Iyengar Yoga, Jivamukti Yoga, Kundalini Yoga, Power Yoga, Sivananda Yoga, Viniyoga, Vinyasa Yoga, and Yin Yoga. But variations exist even within these types. For example, while many people associate Ashtanga Yoga with a fairly vigorous series of physical postures, the word *ashtanga* means "eight" in Sanskrit and refers to the "eight limbs" of yoga set forth by the famous sage Patañjali in the *Yoga Sutras*. Today, Hatha Yoga, with its emphasis on postures, health, and physical fitness, signifies what most Westerners think of as yoga.

But yoga is about more than just postures and physical fitness. The same term "yoga" can apply to esoteric and spiritual disciplines, like the three paths of *karmayoga* (Yoga of Action), *jñanayoga* (Yoga of Knowledge), and *bhaktiyoga* (Yoga of Devotion) most notably laid out in the ancient Hindu text the *Bhagavad Gita*. Yoga also counts as one of six orthodox schools of Hindu philosophy.[10] The word itself comes from the Sanskrit root *yuj*, and like the English word *yoke*, it often means "union."[11] With the essential purpose of removing obstacles that block the true self, yoga presents tools that have the power to effect a transformation in one's life through a confluence of forces in the body, mind, and spirit.

It is challenging for me to further define the discipline beyond laying out some of the types and meanings of yoga. As a trained musician and music scholar, but simply a practitioner of yoga and a curious student of its philosophy, I leave the more profound, dizzying, and even controversial question "What is yoga?" for yoga experts to unpack. Yoga scholarship and discourse have blossomed, especially since 2008, with many excellent studies exploring ancient, classical, and medieval traditions and their transformations into modern yoga.[12]

Still, for the purposes of this book, I provide a short yoga primer to offer a bit of context about modern yoga, to establish basic yoga terms and concepts referred to throughout the book, and to describe yoga practice and philosophy in terms of what Iyengar believed it to be. This is crucial to Menuhin's story. As the great guru dedicated his life to his practice and beliefs, these in turn undoubtedly influenced his students and so framed Menuhin's understanding of yoga.

MODERN YOGA

Although Menuhin himself had never heard of yoga before he first encountered it, yoga has been attracting interest in the West since the nineteenth

century (Henry David Thoreau, for example, was drawn to it in 1849[13]).
Swami Vivekananda (1863–1902) is largely credited for bringing the idea
of yoga to the English-speaking West. A spiritual and intellectual giant,
Vivekananda traveled to the US and the UK in the late nineteenth century
to teach and lecture on yoga, including at the Parliament of the World's
Religions in Chicago in 1893. His seminal book *Raja Yoga* (1896) is often
credited as the beginning of what yoga scholars refer to as modern yoga,
which began to take root as both an esoteric philosophy and a postural/
meditative practice. Modern yoga refers to "certain types of yoga that
evolved mainly through the interaction of Western individuals interested
in Indian religion and a number of more or less Westernized Indians
over the last 150 years."[14]

In addition to Vivekananda, others had influence on modern yoga.
The Indian writer and philosopher Jiddu Krishnamurti (who later became
Iyengar's pupil) was named the Theosophical Society's "world teacher" and
was taken under the tutelage of the organization's leader Annie Besant
in England in 1911 (in 1929, Krishnamurti renounced this title). In that
same period, Aleister Crowley (1875–1947), the British occultist and
writer, blended yoga philosophy from Patañjali's *Yoga Sutras* with his own
esoteric ideas in *Book Four* (1913)[15] and later published *Eight Lectures on
Yoga* under the name Mahatma Guru Sri Paramahansa Shivaji. While one
scholar considers Crowley to have been a "fraudulent self-practitioner of
Tantric Yoga," the celebrated poets W. B. Yeats and T. S. Eliot also knew
of Patañjali's *Yoga Sutras* and referred to the text's esoteric ideas in their
own work.[16]

In the 1930s, yoga philosophy centers were founded in both the US
and the UK, including the Vedanta Society of Southern California in Los
Angeles (1930) by Swami Prabhavananda (1893–1976) and a Ramakrishna
Vedanta Centre in London (1934) by Swami Avyaktananda. The health
benefits of yoga postures began to draw attention, especially from mid-
dle-class women in Britain who belonged to fitness organizations that
incorporated the practice, such as Mary Bagot Scott's Women's League of
Health and Beauty and Eileen Fowler's Keep Fit.[17]

Iyengar and Menuhin's relationship rode this wave of yoga activity in
the UK and the US. In fact, most scholars point to Iyengar Yoga as a model
of how modern yoga grew during the 1950s and 1960s.[18] The emphasis
on yoga in adult education in the UK took root when the Inner London
Education Authority (ILEA), an ad hoc local education authority for the
City of London and the twelve Inner London boroughs, began to offer

yoga classes for adults in 1967. By that time, Iyengar had firmly established himself in the West as a leading teacher of modern postural yoga, which emphasized *asana* practice, and in 1969 ILEA ruled that only teachers approved by him could teach yoga classes through the organization.[19]

PATAÑJALI'S *YOGA SUTRAS* AND THE EIGHT LIMBS OF YOGA

Patañjali's *Yoga Sutras* has become the Bible of modern yoga philosophy and practice. Most yoga scholars and students broadly date Patañjali's codification of ancient yoga philosophy and practice to somewhere between the fifth century BCE and fourth century CE, and the revived text articulates what many modern yoga scholars and practitioners understand the discipline to be.[20] While Vivekananda promoted the ancient text as the basis for what he called *raja yoga* in the West, Tirumalai Krishnamacharya (1888–1989), Iyengar's guru, centered the modern theory and practice of postural yoga on the *sutras*. He passed along this focus as a basis for yoga study and practice to his students, including Iyengar. To this day, in the tradition of Krishnamacharya, at the beginning of an *asana* class Iyengar Yoga students chant an invocation to Patañjali (as do other modern yoga schools, such as those established by Srivatsa Ramaswami and K. Pattabhi Jois),[21] who is often represented as a four-armed manifestation of the king of divine serpents Adisesa/Ananta, forming the couch for Lord Vishnu to rest upon. Patañjali's *Yoga Sutras* forms a strong cornerstone for the conception of authentic "classical" yoga—a belief system yoga practitioners often transmit from guru to disciple. This was certainly the case with Krishnamacharya and Iyengar, and the younger yogi especially exerted a strong influence to elevate the *Yoga Sutras* to such an iconic status.[22] It is reasonable to believe that a similar influence transpired between Iyengar and Menuhin.

Patañjali's work conveys a concise and timeless articulation of yoga in the form of 196 terse *sutras*, or aphorisms, organized into four *padas*, or chapters (some texts omit one *sutra* in the third chapter, making a total of 195). The first chapter, *Samadhi pada* (Meditative Absorption), sets up a philosophical context for yoga around the concept of *samadhi*—the state of total awareness and absorption. It defines yoga as "the cessation of movements in the consciousness,"[23] establishes the distractions and obstacles that hinder it, and describes the final result of overcoming such afflictions.

Patañjali's second chapter, *Sadhana pada* (Practice), offers a practical and "action-oriented"[24] guide for the yoga practitioner to still the mind's ceaseless fluctuations. Patañjali first outlines what he calls *kriyayoga*, or Yoga of Action,[25] built on *tapas* (burning zeal and self-discipline), *svadhyaya* (study and reflection), and *isvarapranidhana* (surrender to a God/Higher Power of one's understanding). He distinguishes five *klesas* (obstacles) encountered by the practitioner, namely *avidya* (ignorance), *asmita* (pride/ego), *raga* (desire/attachment), *dvesa* (hate/aversion), and *abhinivesah* (fear of death/clinging to life). Then he identifies the eight limbs of yoga as the means to liberation. Perhaps the most widely known aspect of yoga philosophy, the eight limbs are

1. *yama* (moral injunctions), namely *ahimsa* (nonviolence, harmlessness), *satya* (truthfulness), *asteya* (non-stealing), *brahmacarya* (chastity, religious studentship), and *aparigrahah* (renunciation of unnecessary belongings)

2. *niyama* (fixed observances), namely *sauca* (cleanliness), *santosa* (contentment), and the three key actions of *kriyayoga*: *tapas* (religious fervor, a burning desire), *svadhyaya* (study that leads to the knowledge of the self), and *isvarapranidhana* (surrender to God)

3. *asana* (posture), the limb most often associated with yoga

4. *pranayama* (regulation of breath)

5. *pratyahara* (internalization of the senses toward their source)

6. *dharana* (concentration)

7. *dhyana* (meditation)

8. *samadhi* (absorption of the consciousness in the self)

Many yoga scholars and commentators group these eight limbs into the four outer limbs of *yama*, *niyama*, *asana*, and *pranayama*; the three inner limbs of *dharana*, *dhyana*, and *samadhi*; and a bridge between the outer and inner levels with *pratyahara*. Yet it is important to understand that these eight limbs are not different paths but rather holistically related branches on the same tree of yoga. Patañjali explains the practice and effects of the first five limbs of yoga in the remaining *sutras* of the second chapter. The third chapter, *Vibhuti pada* (Mystic Powers), explains the last three limbs, *dharana, dhyana,* and *samadhi,* and Patañjali describes the *siddhis* (supernatural powers) that one can acquire by practicing yoga. Patañjali's final chapter, *Kaivalya pada* (Perfect Emancipation), the most esoteric of the four, outlines the fulfillment of yoga in the concept of *kaivalya,* variously translated as "liberation," "absolute freedom," and "aloneness."

IYENGAR YOGA

The story of Iyengar's rise is not only about a dedicated and charismatic yogi bursting on the scene before the eyes of an astonished world. It is also part of the story chronicling the rise of modern yoga itself. Iyengar understood his mission to be the teaching of not only the physical practice of yoga but also, crucially, a yoga philosophy rooted in Patañjali's ancient text, the *Yoga Sutras.* In his later years, Iyengar reflected on his life's work and how, along with many of his students, he carried the message of yoga's dimensions "in the form of physical health, mental poise, intellectual clarity, and spiritual solace for millions and millions of people all over the world."[26] To understand the system of yoga as Menuhin did, there is no better place to turn than the book that Menuhin introduced to the world, Iyengar's *Light on Yoga.*

Early Influences

B. K. S. Iyengar (Bellur Krishnamachar Sundararaja Iyengar) was born on December 14, 1918, in Bellur, a small city in the Mysore State (now Karnataka) about one hundred miles from the southwestern coast of India. He was born the eleventh of thirteen children into a poor, religious Brahmin family during the time of the nationalistic struggle for Indian independence from Britain. Although he never became involved in politics, Iyengar identified with neo-Hindu values around social and ethical issues as he embraced the religion of his birth, the South Indian Hindu tradition Srivaishnavism.[27]

Iyengar's childhood and adolescence strongly shaped his yoga teaching method in adulthood. Iyengar's mother fell ill during the 1918 "Spanish" flu pandemic and nearly died while carrying Iyengar,[28] but, miraculously, both mother and child survived. Iyengar was born a sickly child who suffered from bouts of malaria, typhoid, and tuberculosis, and he was not expected to live beyond age twenty. Yet at age fifteen, under the tutelage of his severe yoga guru and brother-in-law Krishnamacharya (the husband of his sister Namagiriamma), Iyengar began to practice for hours every day to heal his weak and stiff body. Iyengar learned from his strict guru to focus on structure, alignment, and physical fitness in his practice. He probably practiced for as many, or more, hours as Menuhin practiced violin as a child prodigy, and one can imagine these two men undergoing a parallel rigorous training in their respective disciplines.

Krishnamacharya, considered to be one of the fathers of modern yoga, was both an accomplished scholar and a dedicated practitioner who exerted a tremendous influence on Iyengar. Krishnamacharya studied *asana* and *pranayama* in his early years with his father and obtained academic degrees in yoga theory and its related philosophy, Samkhya.[29] For more than seven years, Krishnamacharya diligently practiced and studied yoga with his guru Brahmachari in Nepal.[30] In 1918, he departed from his guru's ashram with the charge to teach and spread the message of yoga, and in 1933 he established his own yoga school in Mysore under the maharaja's patronage. Krishnamacharya integrated Western values of physical fitness and training into his yoga teaching and practice, and he may have been the first guru to teach and practice the vigorous and dynamic Vinyasa, or "flow," type of yoga.[31] He also promoted and disseminated yoga by giving palace demonstrations with his students for the royal family, and he authored numerous articles and books on yoga, most notably *Yoga Makaranda* (*The Nectar of Yoga*) in 1934. Dedicated to the maharaja of Mysore, the work was designed to inspire the general reader and amateur practitioner of the time.[32]

From 1934 to 1937, Iyengar's understanding and practice of yoga developed within Krishnamacharya's yoga environment in Mysore, where intense physical practice was coupled with deep mental and spiritual development.[33] During these three years of studying and living with his guru, Iyengar absorbed Krishnamacharya's systematic approach to and conception of yoga, what he later referred to as "a purely traditional yoga" in line with his guru and his guru's guru who "sowed the seed to think and analyze the practical side to bring about further development in this art."[34] Although his training included only the physical aspects of yoga by practicing *asanas* in a sequential manner, applying yoga therapeutically, and giving demonstrations, Iyengar likely also absorbed a devotional centering of the yoga tradition from Krishnamacharya, as the elder guru studied Patañjali's *Yoga Sutras* and practiced *pranayama*.[35]

Development and Growth

Thanks in large part to Menuhin's support, Iyengar perhaps best represents the rise of modern yoga, as he built on his studies and experience with Krishnamacharya while also continuing his guru's charge to teach and spread the message of yoga. Iyengar absorbed his guru's strict and rigorous approach to teaching, even as he expanded yoga's reach beyond his own South Indian world. Much later, he reflected on both his own stern methods and the closed yoga environment in which he was trained:

> In the old days, spiritual knowledge was considered an esoteric subject and jealously guarded by its masters. They were abrupt in their manner and did not think their pupils were deserving enough. . . . You could say that India at that time was engaged in a struggle of political democracy, but I can assure you that spiritual democracy did not exist. Because I am seen as a stern authoritarian teacher, people do not realize how strongly I have in fact reacted against the harsh and secretive regime in which I was brought up. I am open with everything I have learned, and my strictness has really been a passion for precision so that my students should not suffer from the mistakes and hardship that I had to endure.[36]

Iyengar started teaching in 1936, just two years after he began his yoga practice, and in 1937 Krishnamacharya sent him to Pune, where he became a professional yoga teacher. By Iyengar's own account, yoga was all he knew, and he had to build on that to earn a living.[37] He worked ten hours a day to study, understand, and master his *asana* practice, and a silent video made in 1938 captures the brilliance of Iyengar's practice in his early years.[38] Throughout the rest of his life, Iyengar constantly repeated the never-ending cycle of "learning, unlearning, and relearning."[39]

In addition to his studies with Krishnamacharya, Iyengar also assimilated other current yoga practices happening at the time, such as the work of Swami Sivananda of Rishikesh and developments at institutes in Bombay and Lonavala.[40] A medical doctor named Dr. Gokhale taught Iyengar Western medical terms to help explain and disseminate his style of yoga in anatomical terms. Iyengar explained how he acquired such theoretical knowledge about his *asana* practice:

Doctor V. B. Gokhale . . . was a great help to me. He used to give talks, and I used to give demonstrations. Because I could not speak on yoga . . . he said, "The body is known to me. You leave it to me, I will explain very accurately. And you do the poses." Well, it was a really good combination . . . and while he was explaining I started getting anatomical words, which helped me a great deal to develop my subject.[41]

In 1943, Iyengar married Ramamani, whose involvement in yoga helped support his work and practice. Together they had six children, five daughters and one son, and Iyengar taught yoga to his entire family. Ramamani died at the early age of forty-six, and later, in 1975, Iyengar named his yoga institute the Ramamani Iyengar Memorial Yoga Institute (RIMYI) in her honor. His eldest daughter, Geeta (1944–2018), and his son, Prashant (b. 1949), later succeeded Iyengar as codirectors of RIMYI. As of this writing, Iyengar's granddaughter Abhijata (Prashant's niece) has become the younger face and leader of RIMYI, largely overseeing its activities and teaching regularly.

By 1947 Iyengar had achieved some stature and renown as a yoga teacher in Pune, where he developed his approach by conducting regular yoga classes, giving private instruction, and performing yoga demonstrations for important professional and civic organizations.[42] Iyengar often later referred to himself as an artist or as a performer,[43] and Menuhin, as a performing musician, connected with this dimension of his guru's yoga practice when the two began to work together. Beginning in 1948 and continuing for the next twenty years, Jiddu Krishnamurti, the internationally famous Indian philosopher, writer, and speaker, was Iyengar's most famous pupil. In turn, Krishnamurti would come to influence Iyengar's philosophical thinking and perhaps even the yogi's comfort in dealing with Western students like Menuhin.[44] Later, when Krishnamurti came to lecture in Saanen for the Gstaad Menuhin Festival & Academy between 1961 and 1985, he drew Menuhin's interest in attending the philosophical lectures.[45]

In 1952, when Menuhin met his guru, Iyengar had already been teaching for more than fifteen years, refining his conception of yoga and developing the means by which to transmit it to his students. Iyengar viewed the body as his temple and *asana* as his prayers. Through the body he found a pathway to the true self, then he turned his transformation outward to the world to pass on his knowledge and understanding. His educational mission was to lead his students to explore the concrete, physical aspects in the body through *asana* first and then to understand the more abstract aspects of yoga that focus on the mind and soul. He proved that yoga could create a clean place for the *atma* (soul) to live and so be a healing force. Kofi Busia, one of the most experienced teachers and practitioners of Iyengar's method of yoga, summarizes the guru's approach:

> Through his practice and experience he had found the method to provide that clean place. That discovery became the primary focus of his teachings. It was his duty not only to convey his personal experience that growth was indeed possible through yoga, but also to show how to come by that growth. He there-fore had two essential goals in teaching. There was no getting away from the fact that each individual, through due practice and diligence, had to develop himself or herself emotionally, intellectually and spiritually. But he as a teacher could show how this could be done. His duty was to describe spiritual growth as a goal in a clear and systematic way so all could not only see it, but would be motivated to strive for it. . . . That search for clarity on both points was the heart of his teaching.[46]

Iyengar's Light on Yoga *(1966)*

Light on Yoga would become a seminal work about yoga in Europe and among English-language audiences around the world. Similar in intent to Krishnamacharya's *Yoga Makaranda*, *Light on Yoga* aims to reach the general yoga reader by explaining what yoga is within a philosophical/spiritual framework and by illustrating the physical aspects of its practice with photos and descriptions of specific bodily actions. Yet Iyengar's book vastly expanded Krishnamacharya's work in the presentation and expla-nation of the physical practice as well as in setting up the philosophical/spiritual context. He designed a much more comprehensive book to pres-ent yoga as a practice that embraces the dimensions of body, mind, and spirit, organized into an introduction and three parts: *yogasanas* (yoga postures), *bandha* (posture that contracts and controls certain organs or parts of the body) and *kriya* (in this sense, a cleaning process), and *pranayama* (breath control).

The work first lays out the philosophical/spiritual basis of the disci-pline in the thirty-five-page introduction titled "What Is Yoga?" Although one yoga scholar observes how "Iyengar had interpreted the yoga tradition in careful, tentative, and impersonal fashion,"[47] this introduction represents how Iyengar understood yoga in the 1960s and what he intended to transmit to the reader and students. Even in the very first paragraph, Iyengar defines yoga from the Sanskrit *yuj* "meaning to bind, join, attach and yoke," and he cites an author's commentary on the *Bhagavad Gita* that frames this "yoking of all the powers of body, mind, and soul to God."[48] In addition to framing his definition of yoga within the context of the *Gita*, Iyengar largely draws on Patañjali's *Yoga Sutras*, and he explains how in this school of Indian thought "everything is permeated by the Supreme Universal Spirit (*paramatma* or God) of which the individual human spirit (*jivatma*) is a part."[49] Iyengar's musical metaphor of how the "seer/knower" and the "seen/known" become one in yoga was probably not lost on Menuhin: "It is like a great musician becoming one with his instrument and the music that comes from it. Then, the yogi stands in his own nature and realizes his self (Atman), the part of the Supreme Soul within himself."[50] In addition to the *Yoga Sutras*, Iyengar cites other classic philosophical yoga sources in his exposition of what yoga is, including the *Upanishads* (among the most ancient of Hindu texts) and the three major surviving texts on yoga, namely the fifteenth-century *Hatha Yoga Pradipika* by Swatmarama and the (presumed) seventeenth-century manuals *Siva Samhita* and *Gheranda Samhita*.

Based on Patañjali, Iyengar defines the key yoga concept of *citta*, or consciousness, as the collective of mind, intelligence, and ego, and he identifies yoga as the means to still the *vrttis* (fluctuations) in the consciousness. Yet, to Iyengar, the calming of the mind is a means to an end, as he charges the yogi to carry this state out into the world: "Yoga is the method by which the restless mind is calmed and the energy directed into constructive channels."[51] Also drawing on chapter 6 of the *Gita*, Iyengar defines *karmayoga*, which asks practitioners to abandon selfish desires in their work and to accomplish the goals of yoga through the two fundamental actions of *abhyasa* (constant practice) and *vairagya* (detachment, freedom from desire).

Iyengar then maps out the "stages of yoga" squarely within the context of the Patañjali *Yoga Sutras* over the course of the next thirty pages in his introduction. He first summarizes the eight limbs, or stages, then delineates four *margas*, or paths, on which the yogi can travel to their maker and realize their own divinity, namely *karma* (through work and duty), *bhakti* (through devotion to and love of a personal God), *jñana* (through knowledge), and *yoga* (through control of the mind). The remainder of Iyengar's discourse systematically lays out the "science" of yoga according to Patañjali. He summarizes Patañjali's categories of the *citta vrttis* (fluctuations of the consciousness); the *klesas* (obstacles) to quieting them; the nine distractions that span physical, mental, and spiritual dimensions; and the four remedies to these, including the core yogic values of *maitri* (friendliness), *karuna* (compassion), *mudita* (delight), and *upeksa* (disregard).

Perhaps more relevant to this story of Menuhin and Iyengar, the guru also describes the loving and devotional dynamic between *sisya* (pupil) and guru. He emphasizes how a guru "is not an ordinary guide. He is a spiritual teacher who teaches a way of life . . . [and] transmits knowledge of the Spirit."[52] As Menuhin often devotedly referred to Iyengar as his "guru" in his letters and formal messages of endorsement, we can assume he received such spiritual depth of knowledge from Iyengar, along with rigorous instruction in the physical postures.

Finally, Iyengar explains *astangayoga*, or the eight limbs of yoga, and their constituents from Patañjali's *Yoga Sutras* in detail.[53] Whereas Krishnamacharya briefly summarized each limb with only one paragraph in his *Yoga Makaranda*, Iyengar devotes more than twenty pages of his discourse on yoga to explaining the eight limbs. This final section directly represents Iyengar's understanding of the discipline through the body/mind/spirit text of Patañjali, portraying yoga as a physical practice, a philosophical belief system, and a spiritual way of life. In no uncertain terms, he describes *asana* as a way to train and discipline the mind and to gain complete health in body, mind, and spirit. Most importantly (and a theme we will see recur in Menuhin's view of both *asana* and musical performance), Iyengar teaches that the body is but an instrument to attain spiritual liberation and that it is only part of the threefold body/mind/spirit unity: "Where does the body end and the mind begin? Where does the mind end and the spirit begin? They cannot be divided as they are inter-related and but different aspects of the same all-pervading divine consciousness."[54]

Following Iyengar's opening philosophical framework, the work moves on to its well-known and lengthy second part: the thorough and methodical presentation of yoga *asanas*. Iyengar thought that "a good book is better than a bad teacher."[55] For each *asana*, Iyengar systematically provides the Sanskrit name and meaning, outlines step-by-step instructions on the techniques for its performance, and describes its effect on the body.[56]

Written with the goal of helping people who lacked access to a good teacher, Iyengar's book had a tremendous impact on the growth of yoga around the world. His artistic presentation of *asanas*, accompanied by instructions and descriptions framed in Western medical and physical fitness terminology, surely helped to capture the attention of the public. Also, as one yoga scholar has pointed out, Iyengar's approach coincided with the New Age spiritual ethos of the 1960s, which embraced values of body/mind/spirit holistic health, healing, and personal growth.[57] There is no doubt that *Light on Yoga* was the right book at the right time. It not only helped standardize Iyengar Yoga but also ensured that Iyengar had control of his brand. This was crucial for him financially, as he made his living solely from yoga, and was crucial for maintaining his high standards.[58]

MENUHIN'S EMBRACE OF IYENGAR'S TEACHING AND THE
THREE PATHS OF YOGA

Menuhin's foreword to *Light on Yoga* reflects how he absorbed his guru's body/mind/spirit approach to yoga. As Menuhin assimilated his guru's understanding of yoga, his own musical life and work also began to reflect key yoga traits that may be viewed in terms of those described in Patañjali's *Yoga Sutras* and in the *Bhagavad Gita*. From Patañjali's *kriyayoga* come the three characteristics of *tapas* (burning zeal and self-discipline), *svadhyaya* (study and reflection), and *isvarapranidhana* (surrender to a God/Higher Power of one's understanding), while the *Bhagavad Gita* outlines the three yoga paths of *karmayoga* (Yoga of Action), *jñanayoga* (Yoga of Knowledge), and *bhaktiyoga* (Yoga of Devotion).[59] Table 1.1 illustrates the connections between these core yogic concepts, grouped by the three familiar Western dimensions of body, mind, and spirit.

Although in his writings, letters, and lectures Menuhin rarely refers to the philosophy or spiritual teachings of yoga using the exact terms found in Patañjali's *Yoga Sutras* or the *Bhagavad Gita*, I argue that his

Table 1.1. Connections between dimensions of the body, mind, and spirit; the three components of Patañjali's *kriyayoga* and the three yoga paths from the *Bhagavad Gita*.

Dimension	Patañjali *kriyayoga*	*Bhagavad Gita* Yoga Path
Body	*tapas*/burning zeal	*karmayoga*/action
Mind	*svadhyaya*/study	*jñanayoga*/knowledge
Spirit	*isvarapranidhana*/ surrender to God	*bhaktiyoga*/devotion

actions and belief system embraced their universal values in body, mind, and spirit. For example, when Menuhin undertook his quest to understand body mechanics to correct his violin technique, he applied the physical discipline to change, the mental power of self-reflection, and the spiritual willingness to learn from his guru, Iyengar. Referring to his practice as Hatha Yoga, and in his own words explaining his beliefs that echo principles in the first two limbs of yoga—*yama* (universal moral principles) and *niyama* (one's personal principles)—Menuhin said:

> Yoga, if practiced with reverence . . . is a way of keeping the inner and outer self clean. . . . The glory of yoga is that it can lead to an expansion of every kind—physical, mental, and spiritual. . . . Deep breathing, and the extra intake of oxygen, gives full freedom of motion to the joints, but that is only one of the benefits. You cannot breathe quietly if you have any sense of guilt, anxiety, envy, or impatience. The feedback from this is an enhanced ability to control unworthy emotions and motives during the course of the day.[60]

Menuhin's commitment to maintaining physical, mental, and spiritual health radiates from his life's accomplishments. He ultimately believed that artists are a channel for the divine creative spirit, a power also described by the larger yogic concept of *isvara*. And, as yogis surrender their own wants and desires to this Higher Power (*isvarapranidhana*), Menuhin held that his role as a performer was "to inspire the audience to follow him in his devotion, his devotional act."[61] Through this reverential approach to violin performance, aligned with his guru Iyengar's spiritual practice of yoga, Menuhin demonstrates how music and yoga, for him, became one in body, mind, and spirit.

As a man ahead of his time, Yehudi Menuhin was extraordinary not only because he embraced yoga at a time when it was barely known or practiced in the West but also because of the way he integrated yoga into his life and work and embodied yogic principles through his countless achievements. Iyengar recalled how "Menuhin was humble before his [musical] art," with his ego detached from achievements as he practiced his art with great fervor and "fanaticism."[62] Menuhin's artistry, in turn, motivated Iyengar creatively in his own yoga performances while on his "yogic search for the soul."[63] And just as the spiritual and physical aspects of yoga "encouraged [each] other" in Iyengar,[64] Menuhin's musical art and yoga practice were also two sides of the same coin.

Menuhin's Discovery of Yoga

Menuhin's chance discovery of yoga is remarkable, not least because of how much the practice would come to define key aspects of his life for decades to come. He first encountered yoga in July 1951, eight months before meeting Iyengar, during a tour in Auckland, New Zealand, with his sister Hephzibah (see figure 1.1).

While waiting for Hephzibah in a doctor's office one day, Menuhin came across a little book on yoga. He had never heard of yoga before and was immediately fascinated. Menuhin borrowed the book from the doctor and commenced to experiment with the *asanas* (yoga postures) while on tour that week, enjoying the inner quietness derived from the exercises he practiced in solitude[65] and propelled by a quest to understand bodily movements in his violin playing. At the time of his discovery, Menuhin was facing emotional and physical exhaustion following years of a relentless concert schedule, including performances for troops during World War II, and the breakdown of his first marriage. Yoga as a practice seemed to address the woes he was confronting, including critical problems with his

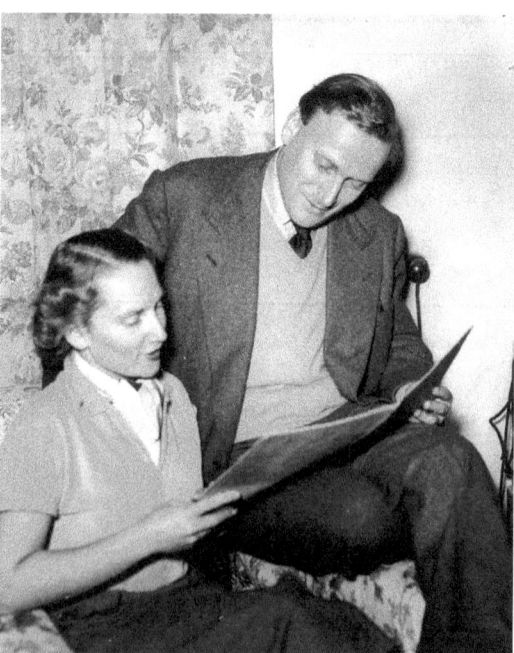

Figure 1.1. Yehudi and Hephzibah Menuhin in Australia 1951. John Oxley Library, State Library of Queensland. Public domain.

body. He writes: "Yoga, whether physical jerks or philosophical system, I had never so much as heard of, but this little introduction to Hatha Yoga—that is the bodily postures, or *asanas*—struck me with the force of revelation."[66] He felt he'd found a path toward solving his problems: "I had stumbled across a key to unlock old enigmas, to make me aware of my capacity, encourage the physical ease missing from my upbringing, point the way to further comprehension of violin playing, and perhaps—if I persevered—stand me on my head in long-delayed fulfilment of childhood ambition."[67] (Head Stand was always Menuhin's favorite pose.)

Inspired by his discovery of yoga, Menuhin began to practice *asanas* on his own for the next seven months. In addition to the pleasure and satisfaction he gained from its practice, Menuhin wanted to prepare himself culturally for his first visit to India, planned for February 1952. There, despite its lack of popularity in the West, yoga was widely practiced. Prime Minister Nehru had invited him to perform on a tour of the country, and in turn Menuhin donated all of his concert proceeds to the Famine Relief Fund (see figure 1.2).

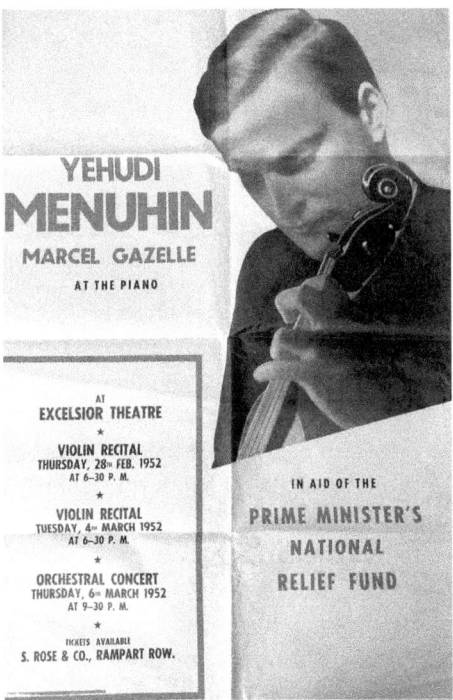

Figure 1.2. Archival poster from Menuhin's first trip to India in 1952. Courtesy of the Foyle Menuhin Archive.

But news of Menuhin's awareness of yoga preceded his arrival. On the musician's first evening in Delhi, Nehru challenged him to demonstrate what he could do. Under the watchful eye of Nehru's daughter Indira (who would succeed her father as prime minister in 1966) and his sister "Nan" Pandit, Menuhin demonstrated his still "somewhat rickety" head stand.[68] The prime minister promptly showed him what a correct head stand should be, and so Menuhin did his best to "emulate his first guru."[69] News of the violinist's interest in yoga and his head stand performance with Nehru spread quickly, and gurus approached Menuhin to offer lessons wherever he went. Menuhin writes, "But not until I met Iyengar, no bearded ascetic, but a good young man with a wife and children, did I take lessons regularly."[70]

After his discovery of yoga, Menuhin sought to practice its principle of union in body, mind, and spirit in his life and work. As it is ultimately concerned with removing obstacles to expose one's true nature, yoga presented a path for Menuhin to regain the effortless way in which he had played the violin as a child. During his lifelong studies with Iyengar, Menuhin practiced what is today recognized as Iyengar Yoga, a style developed through Iyengar's own exploration and rigorous practice of yoga postures and breathing exercises. Menuhin would also spend a great deal of his life promoting the benefits of what he often called Hatha Yoga to others, and he would notably accelerate its spread from India to the West.

Disciple and Guru

It is sometimes said that "when the student is ready the teacher appears," and surely this was the case with Menuhin and Iyengar. In yoga, as with many other Eastern disciplines, aspirants surrender to the teachings of a guru. More than just a teacher, a guru signifies a reverential figure who leads a disciple on a spiritual path from the "darkness" of ignorance to the "light" of knowledge. (In Sanskrit *gu* means "dark" and *ru* means "the remover of that.") While the typical Westerner's spirit of independence and self-determination often prevents such submission, Menuhin knew the importance of master teachers from his own musical training, particularly the mentorship of the renowned Romanian violinist, conductor, and composer Georges Enesco. Just as he was a disciple of Enesco in his musical work, Menuhin became a disciple of Iyengar in his yoga practice. Iyengar would go on to serve as Menuhin's guru for the next four decades and play a powerful role in his career. As Iyengar's son, Prashant, would later observe about Menuhin:

Menuhin had a fascination for eastern mysticism. He was drawn toward the *sadhus* [ascetic mendicants who have renounced the worldly life] and eastern mystics. He had gone far beyond the physical and physiological benefits of practice. He perhaps had *samskara* [imprints from *karma*]. He had a different perception of the world. A common Westerner at that time would not have been fascinated by the things he was fascinated by. He had a fascination for many things that were Indian. Menuhin found that when he met Iyengar. Then, he diligently practiced and applied what he learned.[71]

Soul Connection

When they met in 1952, Menuhin and Iyengar were in their mid-thirties (thirty-six and thirty-four, respectively) and still on the ascendant in their lives—Iyengar in his yoga work and Menuhin in his post–World War II musical career. Born two years apart, the men were contemporaries who possessed core similarities in creative brilliance and determined personalities. They transcended their different East/West cultural backgrounds and connected deeply on personal, artistic, and spiritual levels. Iyengar viewed yoga as "an art, a science, and a philosophy" and believed it "touches the life of man at every level, physical, mental, and spiritual."[72] Menuhin, too, viewed musical performance as a multidimensional art form, where "the performing violinist continually reviews the hours, days and weeks preceding a performance, charting the many elements that will release his potential . . . he knows that when his body is exercised, his blood circulating, his stomach light, his mind clear, the music ringing in his heart . . . then—he is in command."[73] The meeting of these two like-souls ignited a dynamic that would impact each of their individual lives and work. More broadly, their relationship set forces into motion that would influence their respective disciplines of music and yoga. Iyengar accepted Menuhin as a student, and the violinist in turn helped launch Iyengar's international teaching career. Menuhin introduced his guru to the West, and Iyengar eventually became one of the most important yoga teachers in the world.[74]

Immediately after Menuhin first encountered yoga in 1951, he began to practice Hatha Yoga on his own and even found a yoga teacher in the States. But not until he met Iyengar in 1952 would Menuhin begin to cultivate yoga more profoundly in his life and work. After that historic meeting, two strong forces propelled him forward in the discipline: his own regular practice and his teacher-student relationship with Iyengar. Even after just two sessions Menuhin knew Iyengar was the teacher for him, and he was eager to continue learning. Menuhin wrote his first letter to Iyengar later on the very day they met, following up on their earlier conversation in a somewhat authoritative and demanding tone. Writing from the Government House in Bombay, he said: "Pursuant to our conversation of this morning this is to confirm our arrangement whereby you will spend next summer at my home in California. I am wishing for the months of June, July, August, and September."[75] Menuhin offered to pay airfare, board, and lodging, along with a salary of one hundred dollars per month, in exchange for Iyengar teaching yoga to him, his family, and his guests.

Menuhin didn't yet know with whom he was dealing, and judging from the musician's follow-up letter, Iyengar must have clearly replied that this arrangement was not going to work for him. Menuhin took a more conciliatory and humble tone two days later, saying that he understood Iyengar's need for quiet reflection on his request. In a patient manner written with respect to an equal, he assured Iyengar that he understood and would await an answer and "relieve whatever difficulties seem to interfere."[76] Indeed, this was wishful thinking by an overzealous new convert to yoga who seemed to presume that Iyengar would gladly drop his life and work in India to come to the United States as Menuhin's private guru. As it turned out, Iyengar's trip to California never materialized, but their initial sessions and communication established the basis for a relationship of equals. Menuhin was not to be the world-class violinist who engaged Iyengar in his service. Rather, Iyengar decided on his own when and where to take on Menuhin as a student.

Iyengar too recalled the impact of his first meeting with Menuhin. He described treating Menuhin with *shanmukhi mudra* (a yogic gesture that covers the eyes, nose, and ears to quiet the senses) in *savasana* because Menuhin was very tired and full of stress. Iyengar covered the violinist's eyes with his own hands, "taming them, calming them—they seemed to be on fire."[77] Then, after Menuhin woke up fully rejuvenated, he asked for a demonstration. In turn, the guru asked him to show what yoga poses he could do, and Menuhin demonstrated his own head stand. "When I told him that this was not *sirsasana* and corrected him, he immediately felt light in the body."[78] With such potent results, Menuhin was sold. Iyengar taught him twice daily, in the morning and evening, for the next four days (see figure 1.3).

The emotional and physical problems that Menuhin had been suffering since World War II had deteriorated his violin technique. While to

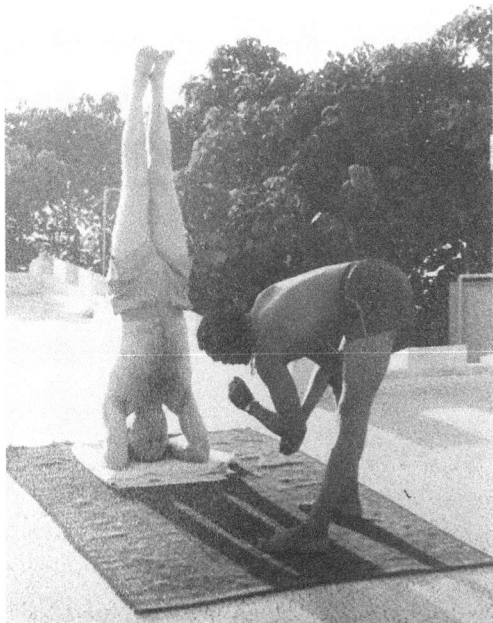

Figure 1.3. Menuhin in *sirsasana* (Head Stand Pose) with Iyengar instructing in Bombay, 1952. Courtesy of the Foyle Menuhin Archive.

my knowledge Menuhin himself never used the word "breakdown" when recounting his postwar struggles, Iyengar did. The yoga master sensed a deep disturbance within Menuhin, noting that the violinist had suffered a "nervous breakdown" prior to 1952 and that his right hand (his bowing hand) would often hurt.[79] Iyengar's insight into the state of Menuhin's mind and spirit during their first meeting illustrates his powerful intuition to read and help people and how deeply the two men connected.

Menuhin's Yoga Training

Archival materials at the Foyle Menuhin Archive at the Royal Academy of Music in London and at RIMYI in Pune, India, provide an extensive portrait of Menuhin's relationship with Iyengar. The Menuhin Archive houses a vast amount of material collected by Menuhin, his family, and his support staff through the years. The contents of the box marked "yoga" document Menuhin's life in yoga and connection to Iyengar through letters, photos, and newspaper clippings. The RIMYI "Menuhin binder" contains thirty-three letters and other documents from Menuhin to Iyengar spanning forty-six years. Their letters range from scribbled notes, hand written when both men were in their thirties, to the formal letters of their later years, typed on the letterheads of the distinguished Lord Menuhin in England and the revered guru Iyengar in India.

The correspondence between Menuhin and Iyengar reveals an especially deep relationship for about fifteen years between 1954 and 1969. Iyengar traveled to Europe during the summers on Menuhin's behalf. In turn, whenever Menuhin traveled to India (he made four trips between 1952 and 1969), "he [Iyengar] would be there throughout the stay to put me daily through my paces."[80] In the 1970s and beyond they saw less of each other as they became more absorbed in the demands of their own careers—Menuhin's as a performer, teacher, and humanitarian and Iyengar's as one of the most influential yoga gurus of the twentieth century. Yet the two men sustained a deep relationship, and they continued to communicate until just a few months before Menuhin's death in March 1999.

In April 1954 Menuhin returned to India to perform in Bombay, Calcutta, Madras, and New Delhi, donating the proceeds from his concerts to Indian charities, as he had done during his first tour in 1952. By this time, Menuhin had fallen in love with all things Indian, ranging from clothing styles to philosophy to music. When asked what made him come back to India, Menuhin replied, "We loved it so much last time, we couldn't stay away," and he described the most outstanding thing about the country as the people's "moral quality, their knowledge of reality and of eternity."[81] The violinist's interest in yoga was by now widely known. One newspaper following his tour reported how Menuhin startled a music critic when he said, "I can do without practicing the violin but I can't do without my yoga exercises."[82]

Menuhin began his lessons in earnest with Iyengar on this second trip to India, and their relationship solidified. Iyengar toured with the violinist for a month to give him yoga lessons, and he recalls how "all the concerts were grand successes."[83] Subsequent correspondence from 1954 reflects a strong relationship of mutual respect and admiration, and they fondly address each other as friends. Menuhin was already realizing the positive impact of yoga on his violin playing, and he was eager to bring Iyengar to Europe so they could continue their work together. With the new salutation "Dear Friend Iyengar," which Iyengar later reciprocated, Menuhin wrote in a personal and humble voice from England: "As you can well imagine, not a day passes but that you are in my mind through the exercises which I continue to perform. I found them of great benefit and am writing you now in the hope that we can arrange to meet before I return to India in two years."[84] This visit to India didn't materialize.

The two men next met in Europe during the summer of 1954. With their firmly established warm and equal relationship, and Menuhin's eagerness to continue working with Iyengar on the yoga poses he found so beneficial, Menuhin invited Iyengar to teach him and his family in Gstaad, Switzerland, for six weeks beginning in August 1954. Menuhin had rented a chalet there as a summer refuge for himself and his family, and three years later he would establish his now renowned music festival in the town. But during that first summer in Gstaad, Menuhin was hoping to "ensure [his] good form for the subsequent eight months tour,"[85] which was to begin on October 1.

The Foyle Menuhin Archive holds many clean reprints of a series of photographs, taken by Jacques Naegeli at the Gstaad Palace Hotel during this visit in 1954,[86] that illustrate exactly what kind of poses Menuhin was learning from his guru. They reveal his impressive accomplishments as a student, even after just a few years of studying, and how serious Menuhin was about his yoga practice. Figures 1.4a1, 1.4a2, 1.4b1, 1.4b2, and 1.4c show examples of Menuhin imitating Iyengar and Iyengar demonstrating an advanced yoga pose.

Menuhin benefitted tremendously from these yoga lessons with Iyengar. He began to work through the technical problems of his aging body and to reconnect with the more intuitive playing methods that he had begun to lose. Through his daily practice, yoga became as integral a part of his life as practicing his violin, and Iyengar later reflected, "Whatever techniques I gave, he used all of them in playing his violin."[87] One of the most famous stories from these early years of their relationship tells how Menuhin viewed Iyengar as his "best violin teacher." Iyengar recalls the impact of that summer: "In appreciation of what yoga had done for him, he [Menuhin] presented me with an Omega wrist watch. At the back of it was the inscription, 'To my best violin teacher, B. K. S. Iyengar. Yehudi Menuhin, Gstaad, Sept. 1954.' His later recitals showed the benefits he derived from yoga. Contact with Menuhin was a great inspiration to me and we regard our meeting as one of the great events of our lives."[88]

Iyengar finally arrived back home in Pune from his European trip, which included a final stop in Paris on October 28. Soon after he had recuperated from his long journey, Iyengar expressed his deep gratitude

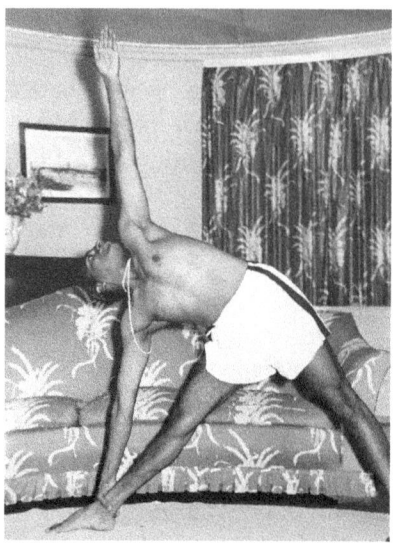

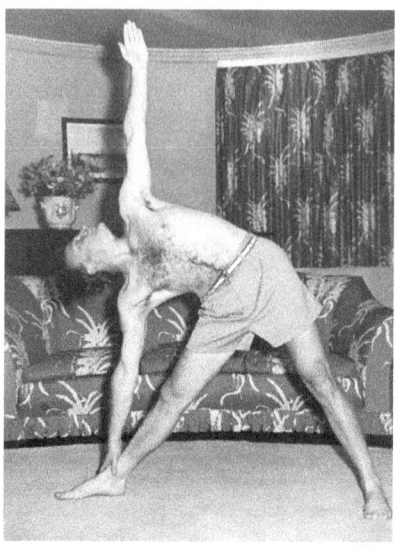

Figure 1.4a1. Iyengar in *trikonasana* (Triangle Pose).

Figure 1.4a2. Menuhin in *trikonasana*.

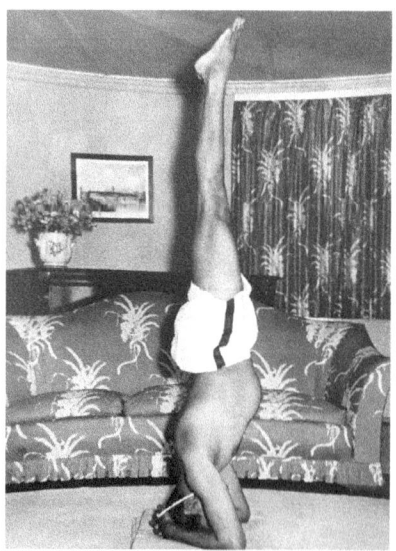

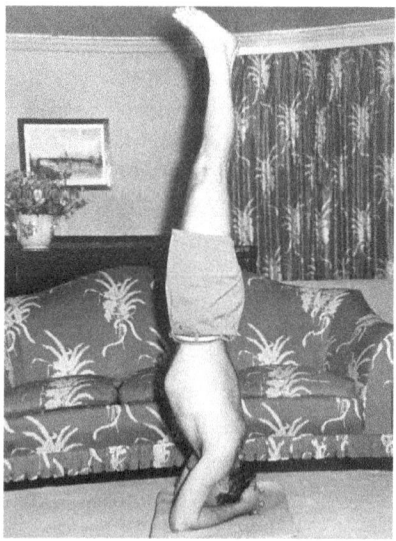

Figure 1.4b1. Iyengar in *sirsasana*.

Figure 1.4b2. Menuhin in *sirsasana*.

Figure 1.4. Iyengar and Menuhin in various yoga poses in Gstaad, 1954. Photos by Jacques Naegeli. Courtesy of Studio Naegeli.

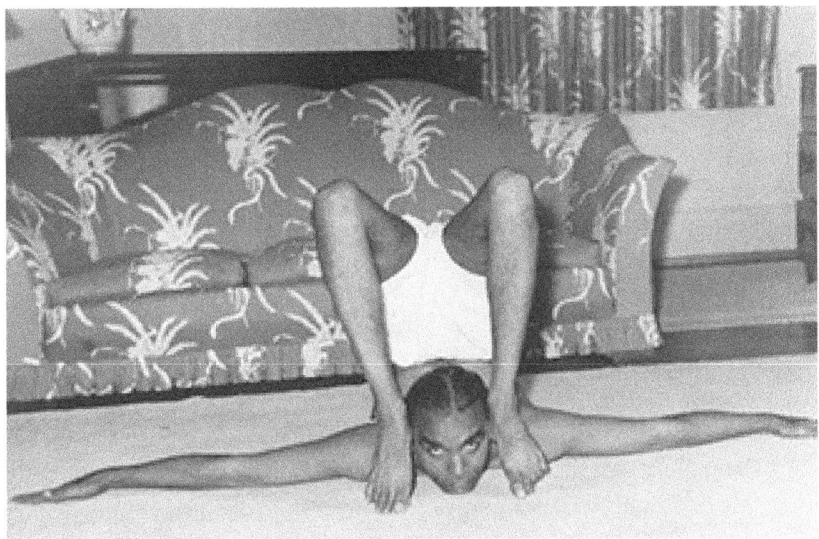

Figure 1.4c. Iyengar in *ganda bherundasana* (Formidable Face Pose).

to Menuhin for taking such good care of him and treating him like family in Gstaad, and he captured the essence of their spiritual, even karmic, connection: "I felt as though my soul moved with you [after Menuhin left Gstaad]. . . . Our love is inseparable now. It is my duty to help you whenever occasion arises."[89]

Menuhin and Iyengar's friendship solidified following their work together in the summer of 1954. As Menuhin deepened his regular yoga practice, he saw immediate effects in his violin playing. He gratefully wrote to his guru that winter: "Not only did I derive pleasure from a better command of my body, but I can assure you that it has a direct expression in my performance on the violin. I have never enjoyed [such] good concerts, or as much control over my violin playing as I do now: much of that is your merit."[90] In hopes of Iyengar's return in 1955 (which didn't happen), Menuhin advised his guru of his tentative concert schedule the following summer.

Iyengar continued to strengthen his role of mentor and spiritual advisor as he encouraged Menuhin in his yoga practice. He wrote to Menuhin in Los Gatos, California, in 1955: "It is your sincere faith in the science and regular practice which is keeping you up physically and mentally. . . . Your nice letter speaks to the nobility of your heart . . . let your music play also loving peace to many."[91] In a letter dated June 1, 1955, Iyengar further articulated the deep soul and karmic connection between them. Inspired by and grateful to Menuhin, he expressed how the violinist's efforts to help people know and understand yoga strengthened his own humble resolve, and more deeply, he saw Menuhin's capacity to bring his music out into the world to heal the hatred and divisions between people:

> As you write, I am though far yet very near you. We meet moment to moment in our heart. I am certain that the way you worked last summer with me in yoga is sure to work on you physically, mentally, and spiritually a great deal. . . . I am happy to know you are practicing regularly. . . . God has to give me strength & courage to carry on my work whatever shortcomings come my way. Your meeting & cooperation has [sic] added more faith in my practice of yoga. It is the will of God that brought us nearer. After all I am not worth the dust even. Through you and your endeavors only the science of yoga will be respected and rewarded. I cannot repay all the good you have done to me. I only pray to God to help me to be grateful & humble to you till the end of this life. Let me pray for your success and let people forget the diversities of hatred against each other and enjoy the one & only sound the music in you & in your instrument & be nearer God.[92]

This connection between Menuhin and his guru Iyengar must have been a fortifying influence during a pivotal time in Menuhin's life. In the mid-1950s, as he transitioned from the famous child prodigy into his adult career, Menuhin began to assert himself as a humanitarian, as in 1956 when he took a stand against apartheid in South Africa. Furthermore, his spiritual connection to yoga and India opened the door to Menuhin's exploration of Indian music, performances of which he would include as the impresario and organizer of music festivals, both in Switzerland and in the UK.

Menuhin continued his efforts to bring Iyengar to Switzerland and the UK in the years ahead. Looking for a new center of residence away from California, the Menuhins—including Yehudi and his second wife, the British dancer Diana Gould (1912–2003); their two sons, Gerard and Jeremy; and his daughter Zamira by his first wife Nola Nicholas[93]—moved from America to Europe in 1955. Menuhin rented a chalet in Gstaad as the family's headquarters from April 1956 to April 1957 and settled in the Highgate district in London in 1959. By July 1960 they established a more permanent center in Gstaad by building their own summer home. Since Iyengar was part of the Menuhin family during those summers together in Gstaad, yoga classes also included the children.

The year after Iyengar's first trip abroad in 1954, Menuhin wrote in the fall of 1955 how he hoped "to repeat the pleasant summer [they] had last year"[94] as he laid down stronger roots in Gstaad. During the summer of 1956, Menuhin began to enlarge the circle of prospective students and financial supporters for his guru among his friends and colleagues in the Swiss town. That same year, Iyengar made his first trip to the US on the invitation of Rebekah Harkness, the heiress of the Standard Oil Company. Menuhin had introduced the two, and Iyengar gave her private yoga lessons and also performed demonstrations in New York and Washington, DC.[95]

Menuhin's work with Iyengar in the summer of 1956 served him especially well as he embarked on his fall 1956 tour. He had been experiencing back pain for some time, and it became so intolerable while in South Africa that he opted for surgery.[96] He credited yoga for his strong recovery as he rather sheepishly confided the details of the laminectomy with fusion to his guru: "Dear Friend: In a way, I feel ashamed to write to you from my present condition, but on the other hand, if it were not for the yoga exercises I did last summer I would hardly have been able to survive the weeks preceding the operation, nor to come out of it with such flying colours."[97]

Menuhin's third trip to India early in 1962, part of an international tour with his sister Hephzibah, further strengthened his relationship with Iyengar as he was able to make time to connect and train with his guru. Menuhin's performance schedule in India, which included a concert in memory of Gandhi, also supported efforts to raise funds for those in need, including the Poona [Pune] Relief Fund and the sufferers of Bihar, per Iyengar's suggestion.[98] While planning this visit with Iyengar, Menuhin promised to set aside time to meet an Indian violinist (most likely Prashant's teacher) and indicated he was looking forward to seeing Iyengar's manuscript for a book on yoga. To document his own yoga progress, Menuhin excitedly reported in a postscript: "I am continuing my exercises and feel I have never done them on my own as well as I am doing them now. I am beginning to balance on my hands and beginning to do the back bend, when the carpet is not too slippery!"[99]

During this visit, Menuhin and Iyengar further deepened their soul connection. Menuhin recommended Iyengar's passport renewal to Indian government officials, and he eloquently extolled the virtues of Iyengar as "one of India's most precious exports [who] commands the devotion and gratitude of countless people in England, Europe, and the USA—people from the most distinguished to the simplest—who recognize in him the surest exponent of one of India's most prized arts—that of Hatha Yoga."[100] The Iyengar family warmly received Menuhin into their home for dinner on this visit, after which Menuhin immediately sent a humble thank you note to Mrs. Iyengar on Raj Bhavan hotel stationary. With his characteristic gracious charm, Menuhin wrote, "How can I possibly express how deeply touched I am by your fervent and selfless generosity—for I know not only to appreciate the art which is your cooking but the infinite effort and work, the patience and trouble you took to prepare the magnificent banquet of last night?"[101]

Iyengar's son Prashant was twelve at the time of Menuhin's 1962 visit. The violinist made a huge impression on Prashant, and he recalls when Menuhin visited Iyengar's classes in Mumbai. "Students performed for him and one of Guruji's students, Minoo Choi, stayed in *sirsasana* for the entire time—maybe 45 minutes to one hour. Then, we cut a cake shaped like a violin. Our fascination as children at that time was to see 'a foreigner.'"[102] (Menuhin's concert with Hephzibah also made a strong impact on Prashant. He and his sister imitated the Menuhin duo, where Prashant "played" the violin with two sticks and she mimicked the piano on a trunk. This ignited Prashant's interest in music and the violin, and he "started learning Hindustani classical music but played it in the Western style."[103]) Seeing his son's interest in music, Iyengar enrolled him in violin lessons with a local violinist, Professor Upadhyay, and a few years later bought him a violin while in London with the help of Menuhin.[104] Menuhin continued to take an interest in Prashant's musical progress. Whenever the young musician would send recordings of himself playing Indian ragas (the melodic framework for improvisation in Indian music) in "Western tones," Menuhin always replied with encouraging letters.[105] In a 1963 letter, Menuhin responded to an update from Iyengar about Prashant with yoga-like references to *tapas*, writing he was happy to learn his "young colleague" was "fired with devotion and ambition and is working at his violin with enthusiasm."[106] Later, during his fourth trip to India in 1969, Menuhin presented a Stradivari violin to Prashant and attended his recital. Naturally, Menuhin also continued to take yoga lessons with Iyengar.

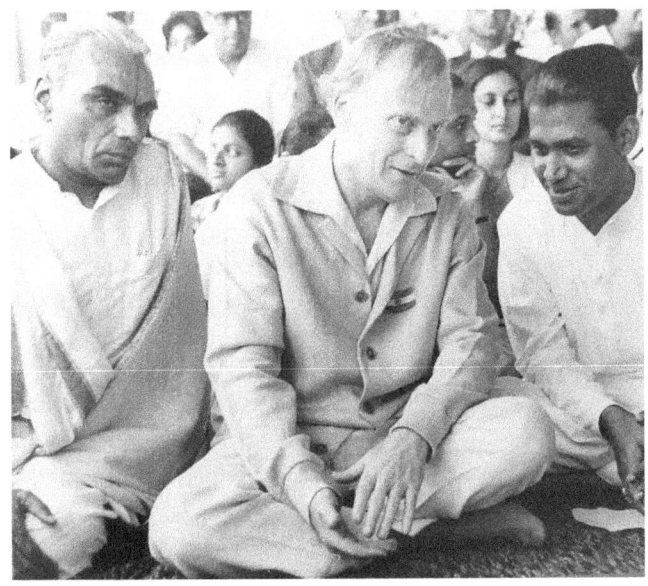

Figure 1.5. Prashant Iyengar's student violin recital in Bombay, 1969. Courtesy of the Foyle Menuhin Archive.

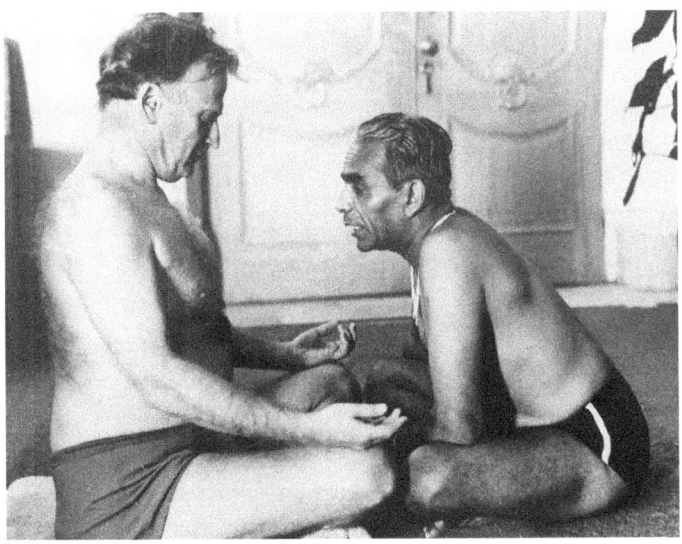

Figure 1.6. Menuhin and Iyengar lesson in Bombay, 1969. Courtesy of the Foyle Menuhin Archive.

After they left India on the 1962 tour, Yehudi and Hephzibah Menuhin performed in New Zealand and Australia. Menuhin's muscles and tendons "had not yet consolidated all the good work" Iyengar had given him during their visit, and although his "strength and swing from the feet was wonderful," he strained his right hip and the side of his back in "enthusiastic exuberance."[107] Menuhin visited a good "physical medicine man in Auckland and another later in Melbourne," and he happily reported to his guru from Melbourne that his tissues had recovered so that he could practice yoga again: "I am *much* more flexible and strong (have even done some standing poses) than I was before I came to India and I do the shoulder stand nearly vertically, also the combination exercise [?] is very good—I balance for a few seconds on my hands [handstand]—and put my head on my knees [forward fold] as never before."[108] Menuhin proposed plans for their next meeting in the summer and hoped to please his teacher: "If we do have a chance to meet in London *before* Gstaad you will I am sure find me in good shape."[109]

Menuhin finished out the year back home in London following a strenuous tour in Russia. He found it difficult to keep up his yoga practice there, and he felt the consequences, despite a five-day rest at the Bircher Clinic in Zurich. He admitted to Iyengar: "I did not keep up my exercises as well as I would have liked to in Russia: the floors were too dirty for one thing and that is no doubt one reason why I came back particularly battered. But I am restored again, and I think you would not be too displeased with me."[110] It seems Iyengar had a premonition about Menuhin's difficult trip and had written Menuhin about a dream he had. Menuhin wrote how he was touched that Iyengar "should have dreamed of Diana [Menuhin's wife] and me. Actually, we did have a terribly grueling time during our month's tour of Russia."[111]

Menuhin's Role in Iyengar's *Light on Yoga*

Menuhin and Iyengar's letters also reveal the reciprocal nature of their relationship during the 1950s and 1960s. During these most intensive years of working together, Menuhin promoted his guru and Indian culture in the West while he diligently studied and practiced yoga with Iyengar. Iyengar's important work *Light on Yoga*, with the foreword written by Menuhin, especially merits a detailed examination in light of Iyengar's influence on Menuhin.

For a number of years, Iyengar had been working on the comprehensive book detailing his approach to yoga designed to reach aspiring yoga students who didn't have access to a good teacher. During a trip to Europe in 1960, Iyengar had brought the manuscript and photo prints for the project with him from India in hopes of finding a London publisher. He left the manuscript with Menuhin in London for help with any mistakes and wording in the text. Menuhin was to bring the manuscript with him to Gstaad when they met there later that summer.[112]

Meanwhile, Menuhin worked his publishing contacts to help Iyengar with his book. While in Gstaad, he sent Iyengar's manuscript to John "Jock" Murray in London, assuring him Queen Elisabeth of the Belgians, another famous student of Iyengar's, would also endorse it.[113] Interestingly, as Menuhin sought advice about prospective publishers for Iyengar, he also described typical book woes for authors struggling with their first publication. In Iyengar's case, this entailed working with a prospective publisher in India who had encouraged him to write the book but had not helped with the expenses or given him a contract.

Iyengar's *Light on Yoga*, which was eventually published in 1966, not only clearly articulates Iyengar's approach to the physical practice and teaching of yoga but also reveals his understanding of the deeper dimensions of yoga in mind and spirit. One can imagine that Menuhin, in turn, absorbed his guru's holistic physical, philosophical, and spiritual conception of yoga as articulated in this book. Iyengar and Menuhin approached their respective disciplines with the same rigor. Iyengar's systematic and methodical approach to teaching yoga, which he documented and expressed in *Light on Yoga*, was perfectly suited to Menuhin's quest for understanding the mechanics of good violin playing. Iyengar's emphasis on body alignment and clarity of instruction in the practice of *asana*, coupled with the belief that the physical practice penetrates to deeper levels of the mind and the soul, surely appealed to Menuhin's conviction that he would have to employ his intellect as well as intuition to achieve mastery of the violin. As he wrote, "Intuition was no longer to be relied on; the intellect would have to replace it,"[114] and the path Iyengar laid out for his students surely guided Menuhin toward accomplishing this goal.

Menuhin's foreword to *Light on Yoga* reflects how he absorbed his guru's body/mind/spirit understanding of yoga. It both encapsulates how he understood yoga as a holistic practice and endorses Iyengar as a foremost yoga master.[115] Menuhin employs musical metaphors to describe how the body is "our first instrument, we learn to play it, drawing maximum resonance and harmony." Drawing on experience from his own practice over the previous fifteen years, Menuhin points to how the body connects to the mind because our attitudes in life have physical counterparts in the body. In order to correct these attitudes, we must first align our bodies. In the spiritual dimension, he writes how we learn about "continuity and a sense of the universal" from the alternation of tension and release in "eternal rhythms" of inhalation and exhalation, "which in turn teach us the cycles, waves, and vibrations of the universe." Menuhin praises Iyengar's method for how it prevents physical and mental illness, protects the body, and develops self-reliance and assurance. He finally links yoga to the universal laws of respect for life, truth, and patience, since all are required to quiet the breath, calm the mind, and firm up the will. He humbly concludes: "If this book will serve to spread this basic art and will ensure that it is practiced at the highest level, I shall feel more than ever grateful for having shared in its presentation."

Considered by many today to be the Bible of yoga, *Light on Yoga* has been translated into twenty-six languages and has had numerous printings. With this great achievement, Iyengar accomplished his mission to bring yoga out into the world. The book was an enormously successful inaugural work, and its impact has continued for decades. After the publication of *Light on Yoga*, Iyengar, like Menuhin, became a prolific writer (Iyengar's second and third major books, *Light on Pranayama* and *Light on the Yoga Sutras*, are discussed in Chapter 3). Iyengar had little formal education and received great assistance from others. In the case of *Light on Yoga*, he received research and editorial assistance from his student B. I. Taraporewala and the British editor Gerald Yorke.[116] While Yorke was influential in publishing earlier books on yoga in Britain, including such titles as *Heaven Lies Within Us [On Yoga]* (Bernard, 1941), *Hatha Yoga* (Bernard, 1950), and *Yoga and Health* (Yesudian and Haich, 1953),[117] none have made the lasting impact of *Light on Yoga*.

Later Relationship

Menuhin and Iyengar continued their close connection and correspondence in support of each other through the rest of the 1960s. As a result of Menuhin's introductions, Iyengar Yoga continued to grow tremendously both in the UK and on the European continent. It became especially strong in Switzerland, as Iyengar voyaged to the country regularly to teach Menuhin in Gstaad until 1972. By that year, Iyengar had already visited Switzerland thirteen times, and he later returned in 1986, 1990, and 1997 to teach in the Swiss cities Basel, Bern, and Zurich.[118] The nearby Menuhin Center Saanen, officially established in 2003 after its director Rolf Steiger spent years collecting souvenirs, programs, clippings, and photos from Menuhin's life and the Gstaad Festival, celebrated fifty years of yoga in Switzerland in conjunction with the Iyengar Yoga Vereinigung Schweiz (Iyengar Yoga Swiss Union) in 2004. This special anniversary event commemorated the unique bond between Menuhin and Iyengar by highlighting Menuhin's lessons with his guru, Iyengar's first official demonstration in the Landhaus in Saanen in 1962, and the spread of Iyengar yoga throughout the country.

While the publication of *Light on Yoga* in 1966 marked a pivotal point in Iyengar's ascending career, the guru was already becoming more well-known internationally. In the fall of 1965 Menuhin noted his guru's rising impact when he replied to a recent letter from Iyengar to express gratitude for their summer activities and to comment on how touched he was to read how much Iyengar helped the Belgian Queen Elisabeth. More profoundly, Menuhin reflected on how deeply she, and all of Iyengar's students in Europe, care for him: "I know just how she felt when she saw you go, and probably realized that she might not see you again. [In fact, the Queen Mother died two months later on November 23, 1965]. If only you could duplicate yourself and there were several of you about, we would all be much better for it. Perhaps your children?"[119]

Menuhin's status in England was also rising. In recognition of his artistic accomplishments, Menuhin was made an honorary Knight of the British Empire (KBE) in 1965, and he would become Sir Yehudi upon assuming British citizenship in 1985. Over the course of the next several decades, all the way until his death, Menuhin sustained his connection with Iyengar, although time and scheduling constraints limited their in-person meetings. Their correspondence also became more intermittent, as it centered mostly around milestones achieved in their respective lives from the 1970s to the 1990s. Still, Menuhin's ongoing commitment to maintaining the relationship with his guru until his final years highlights how thoroughly he had integrated yoga into his life and the remarkable role that this friendship had in Menuhin's life and yoga practice.

Menuhin's milestone birthday messages to Iyengar reflect his ongoing respect for the guru. For example, his message for Iyengar's sixtieth birthday souvenir book in December 1978 echoes some of his views on yoga expressed in the foreword to *Light on Yoga*, especially on the mind/body connection: "The study of Yoga over the years has convinced me that most of the fundamental attitudes to life have their physical counterparts in the body."[120] Even as he held up Iyengar as a model teacher so desperately needed by humankind, Menuhin had not lost sight of his guru as an artist: "I cannot praise too highly the beauty of Mr. Iyengar's art, his precision and refinement."[121] Two years later, as he was recuperating from an illness, Menuhin reported to Iyengar about the ongoing benefits of his daily morning yoga practice and how "head stand, plough-pose, shoulder-stand and general mobility is good, especially as I apply what I learn to practicing the violin and to walking . . . I feel I am still successfully climbing, as I can play better now than ever before."[122]

As Menuhin paid tribute to his guru on his seventieth birthday in December 1988, he reflected on how deeply Iyengar had influenced his life: "As a dedicated teacher, precise, observant, perfectionist, and buoyed by a sense of obligation to and responsibility for humankind, he [Iyengar] was a modelling influence in shaping a form of holistic awareness of mind and body, an impression that has continued to act both consciously and sub-consciously upon my well-being—my daily routine, which, since our summers together, I have further tailored to specific needs and schedules."[123]

Menuhin made two additional trips to India in the last decade of his life in the fall of 1995 and in January 1998. Although he corresponded with Iyengar, he was not able to meet his guru in person during either visit. Still, Menuhin dutifully reported on his yoga practice, saying in 1995 that he could stand on his head and do the Plough Pose and Shoulder Stand Pose but could not quite cross his feet onto his thighs like he used to.[124] While there was a misunderstanding and some hurt feelings about a missed opportunity to meet in person that year, their friendship remained intact.[125] According to one of Iyengar's long-term students and a senior yoga teacher in the United States, the two men *did* meet again in London in 1996, and he took a picture of that meeting.[126] I believe this is the last time the two friends saw each other in person.

Menuhin's final tour of India the year before his death was fraught with logistical and organizational problems from the beginning, and a burst of correspondence between Menuhin and Iyengar centered around another missed opportunity to meet. Still, Iyengar wanted to help Menuhin "recharge the battery & your body to do yoga."[127] By this time, Iyengar regularly used props in his practice and teaching (Iyengar was the first to systematically develop the use of props in *asana* practice, and they are now a hallmark of Iyengar Yoga), and he instructed Menuhin to set up two small stools and put his shoulders between them to do head balance with ease and comfort while keeping the head loose. Regarding the correction Menuhin needed for his back, however, Iyengar said he should be there in person.[128]

Remarkably, even in this last year of his life at age eighty-two, Menuhin persevered with his yoga practice. When he expressed interest in trying to do the headstand with props, Iyengar provided further detailed instructions in a follow-up letter along with a photo of himself demonstrating the pose to encourage Menuhin to maintain his head balance.[129] Menuhin was thankful for Iyengar's good advice and began to do his "exercises" again.[130] Iyengar was so delighted that he sent Menuhin a sequence of poses accompanied by illustrative photos to help in his practice. Ever the supportive teacher, Iyengar also sent contact information of his advanced student in Paris named Biria so Menuhin could request that Biria come to London to help him.[131]

Just a few months before his death, Menuhin again connected with Iyengar around the milestone of the guru's eightieth birthday in December 1998. Iyengar had personally requested Menuhin's presence in a letter that signifies how deeply their lives had impacted each other's over the nearly fifty years of friendship, both in terms of the worldwide dissemination of yoga and in their personal soul connection: "As you are the hub of my work in making the subject of yoga reach millions of people in the world, my inner voice is praying that you, as the other half of my soul in the field of yoga, should grace such an occasion so that it is going to be a monumental contact of the ordinary intellectuals of the world with genius like yourself. . . . Without your presence here, the function will be just a soulless function for me."[132] Geeta Iyengar followed up on her father's personal invitation in a formal letter addressed to "Lord Menuhin," where she described how the celebration would honor the great accomplishments of Iyengar and requested Menuhin to send a message.[133]

Since he had been traveling in Romania and elsewhere during that summer, Menuhin did not receive either of these letters from Pune until he returned home early in the fall of 1998. In what I believe to be Menuhin's last letter to his guru, he gratefully acknowledged the photos of *asanas* Iyengar had sent him to practice and praised Iyengar for his originality: "All are very, very useful for your old pupil. What excellent ideas they are, which I will try to put to use. I am very touched by the trouble you have taken to have these practical and infinitely helpful poses made for me . . . [it is] magic how you make use of props to limit the extreme perfection of the perfect pose to allow those imperfect beings to improve themselves."[134] Although Menuhin indicated hopes to give a concert in Bombay in early November and would gladly visit then (sadly, this trip never materialized), he regretted he could only send a short message to include in the eightieth birthday program. Menuhin's final words to Iyengar indicate how he maintained his yoga practice to the end, promising "I shall put your photographs to good use and one day will give you a report. With my love and admiration to you, dear friend, Yehudi Menuhin."[135] Menuhin's message for the great celebration praised Iyengar and conveyed his pleasure about how the birthday festival was to include Indian classical music, dance, and drama. "I hope I have not missed the opportunity of joining my name to the many who have benefitted from B. K. S. Iyengar's gift, if I may say so, mankind. Perhaps no other single person has contributed so much to a real understanding of Hatha Yoga, from India where we first met to the USA, England and many other places as well. . . . As an old admirer and student of Dr. Iyengar, this message comes with all my heart. Yehudi Menuhin."[136]

Iyengar gratefully acknowledged Menuhin's birthday message in what I believe to be his last letter to his renowned student, writing that he hoped they could meet in November.[137] As this late-life correspondence shows, the soul connection first established in the 1950s between the two men remained intact to the end of Menuhin's life only a few months later in March 1999.

As peers in age and stature in their respective fields of music and yoga, Menuhin and Iyengar nurtured a forty-seven-year relationship from their mid-thirties into their early eighties. From their initial meeting in 1952 to their professional collaborations in the 1960s and finally through later correspondence between the 1970s and 1990s, Menuhin and Iyengar inspired each other through their mutual admiration and respect. In turn, the fruits of their deep connection that intersected on artistic, philosophical, and spiritual planes inspired each other through yoga and music.

Once Menuhin encountered yoga and connected with Iyengar, he stayed on his yoga course for the rest of his life. Through his regular yoga practice, Menuhin integrated "his lessons, and the lessons built on lessons [to] evolve into an item on the day's agenda as routine as bathing."[138] His yoga practice bore fruit in the body/mind/spirit dimensions of his life.

He gained a confidence that his musical gift was now under his technical control; he gave back by sharing his knowledge through "the service of music and teaching"; and in the spiritual realm, he deepened his own "general human experience."[139]

Chapter 2

Early Influences and Career

Menuhin's Path to Embracing Yoga

Menuhin exhibited a strong idealism and open-mindedness about the world, both during his childhood and later as a yoga practitioner. His early family life played an important role in laying the foundation for this worldview, while his inherent idealism and culturally inclusive beliefs provided the emotional and spiritual groundwork for his embrace of yoga as an adult. When viewing the early influences and musical career that formed the foundation for Menuhin's remarkably creative and spiritual life, it is really no surprise that he felt so drawn to the practice and discipline of yoga as an adult.

Development as a Classical Performer

EARLY TRAINING

Menuhin was born in New York City on April 22, 1916. His parents, Moshe ("Aba") and Marutha ("Imma") Menuhin had arrived in America as part of the wave of Russian Jewish immigration in the early twentieth century. His mother proudly named him Yehudi, which means "the Jew." As expectant parents looking for their first apartment, Moshe and Marutha suffered from an antisemitic remark by a prospective landlady who assured the couple she didn't take Jews. After this bitter and hostile experience, Marutha vowed their child's name would leave no doubt about his heritage.[1] Menuhin's family moved to San Francisco when he was two, and his younger sisters, Hephzibah and Yaltah, were born in 1920 and 1921, respectively.

Menuhin's family background blended cultural elements from his Russian immigrant parents, including traditions of Hasidic Judaism and esoteric thought. His father was raised in a Hasidic community, and its emphasis on music, dance, and direct mystical experience in turn influenced his son. Moshe was constantly at his son's side, overseeing his concert schedule and travels. Marutha, a talented linguist, took charge of the children's education, which concentrated on languages and transmitted an "exotic elsewhere."[2] Their home-schooled daily activities mainly consisted of practicing music and studying, with breaks for outdoor playtime and family outings organized by Marutha. The tight-knit family sheltered the young Menuhin from the world, and he maintained a kind of childlike innocence throughout his life.

Menuhin began violin lessons at age five and from the beginning displayed extraordinary natural talent. His sisters were also extremely talented. They both become accomplished pianists, and Hephzibah later often performed with her brother. Of the three talented siblings, however, only Yehudi Menuhin attained a successful concert career, perhaps due to the fact that, besides his prodigious talent, he was the only one of the three that his parents pushed and supported on this professional path.

Under the tutelage of Louis Persinger (1887–1966), Menuhin made his public debut in 1924, gave his first full-length recital in San Francisco in 1925, and made his New York recital debut in 1926. In late 1926, the Menuhin family made its first trip to Europe to begin the young prodigy's concert career. He made his Paris debut in 1927 and his Berlin and London debuts in 1929, the year he also returned to Paris. The Menuhin family established homes in New York, Paris, Basel, and Los Gatos, California throughout these years.

His parents kept all concert reviews from him, even though he played to such rave headlines as "The Miracle Boy," "Genius," "Uncle Sam's King David of the Violin," "The Violinist of the Century," and "The Einstein of the World's Virtuoso Violinists."[3] In fact, Albert Einstein, who was an amateur violinist himself, heard the young genius perform at his Berlin debut, with Bruno Walter conducting, on April 12, 1929. After the concert, Einstein rushed backstage to embrace Menuhin. He exclaimed, "Now I know there is a God in heaven," and he reported to the *Musical Courier*, "The talent of the boy is the greatest I have ever observed. The spiritual conception of everything he plays, whether by Bach or Brahms, plus the technical perfection with which he masters a large violin with his little, plump fingers reminds me of my sensations forty years ago when I heard the great Joachim play for the first time."[4] Other luminaries heaped praise on the young virtuoso, including the great Italian conductor Arturo Toscanini, who lauded Menuhin after his New York concert on February 22, 1930, by shouting, *"Bravissimo, Yehudi caro! Bravissimo!"*[5]

Menuhin became a true citizen of the world during his formative years as he toured throughout the United States, Europe, Australia, New Zealand, South Africa, and Latin America. The years 1931–1935 spanned an intensive four-year concert schedule during his adolescence, culminating in 1935 with a demanding performance schedule that included "a total of 110 concerts in sixty-three cities of thirteen different countries."[6] Menuhin later reflected on how these international trips formed his personality: "The twice-yearly transatlantic crossings of adolescence did not split my life in half; rather they linked my double heritage into a seamless whole."[7]

During his very first trip to Europe, the young Menuhin also encountered the first inklings of the physical struggles with his instrument that would continue throughout his life and become one of the catalysts for his yoga practice. He admitted to never learning proper violin technique in his early years, producing instead the desired sound through his own intuition and musicality. In 1927 Persinger, his teacher in the States, had arranged for the boy to audition in Brussels for the renowned violinist Eugène Ysaÿe (1858–1931), with whom Persinger had studied. Upon request, Menuhin delivered a flawless performance of Lalo's *Symphonie Espagnole*, as the great maestro accompanied him in pizzicato on his own violin. After his brilliant performance, however, Menuhin struggled terribly when asked to play an A major arpeggio in four octaves. Ysaÿe commented prophetically, "You would do well, Yehudi, to practice scales and arpeggios."[8] This advice would come back to haunt Menuhin in the years ahead, as he embarked on a lifelong quest to gain a deeper understanding of his body in its relationship to his violin playing.

CHILDHOOD MENTORS

Despite his largely sheltered childhood, Menuhin did have important role models outside of his family. During his early life, he was strongly influenced by two brilliant individuals, later describing them as two of the most "evolved people" he ever knew:[9] Willa Cather (1873–1947), a family friend and one of the most famous American authors at the time, and the renowned Romanian violinist, conductor, and composer George Enescu (1881–1955), also known by the French form of his name, Georges Enesco (I will refer to him with this spelling, as Menuhin did).

Known for his works influenced by Romanian folk music, Enesco had come to San Francisco to conduct his own First Symphony and to perform the Brahms Violin Concerto in March 1925. The eight-year-old Menuhin sat in the audience and later described falling under a kind of spell cast by the charismatic and enigmatic musician. He remembered that concert vividly: "Before a note was sounded, he had me in thrall. His countenance, his stance, his wonderful mane of black hair—everything about him proclaimed the free man, the man who is strong with the freedom of gypsies, of spontaneity, of creative genius, of fire."[10] With such a description, Menuhin could have been portraying a yogi.

In Paris two years later, shortly after his audition with Ysaÿe, Menuhin had another opportunity to see Enesco perform. Determined to study with the famous Romanian musician rather than with Ysaÿe, Menuhin went backstage to convince Enesco to give him lessons.[11] Enesco relented to the persistent young violinist, and they arranged for lessons in Paris between tour dates during the following months.

Menuhin remained a disciple of Enesco, and the two violinists would work together and remain friends until Enesco's death. Enesco's impact on Menuhin was notable in shaping not only the young violinist's musical development but also his worldview. Enesco conveyed sheer expression and musicality above technique and theory to Menuhin.[12] He also sparked a love for music of other cultures in his young pupil and so planted a seed for Menuhin's later fascination with Eastern music. Late in the summer of 1927, Menuhin and his family spent two months in Romania, where the impressionable eleven-year-old began his "lifetime's journey to the East and to the past,"[13] finding great unity between the people and their natural environment. During that trip, Enesco took Menuhin to hear a gypsy violinist, which was the first time Menuhin had heard this style of folk music. Menuhin later described his astonishment at how the fiddler could "fetch such extraordinary sounds from primitive instruments, using bows that were saplings strung with unbleached horsehair."[14] He also heard echoes of the Hasidic melodies that his father sang,[15] and Menuhin came to love what he often referred to as "gypsy music" for its earthiness and passionate freedom of expression.[16] He always fondly associated this music and culture with his Romanian teacher.

Enesco also transferred humility to his young student, a trait that remained with Menuhin all his life as both a musician and a yogi who kept his ego in check. As Robert Magidoff, Menuhin's first biographer, describes: "The one idea Enesco never tired of impressing upon Yehudi was that the performer was at all times the servant of the music; that no great composition was ever written merely as a vehicle for the virtuoso, that greatness lay in giving true expression to the intent and purposes of the composer."[17] Enesco's passionate conception of music and his naturalistic approach continued to inspire and influence Menuhin for the remainder of his life.

Willa Cather (1873–1947), the American author of such renowned novels as *O Pioneers!*, *My Ántonia*, and *One of Ours*, was another important early influence on Menuhin. She became a close family friend of the Menuhins, as their family life often included small gatherings of artists, intellectuals, and writers. Cather played an important role in nurturing Menuhin's ideas of diversity and open-mindedness, which prepared the way for his later embrace of yoga and his lifelong motivation for cultural and musical exchange. To Menuhin, the great author possessed the "unity in diversity" principle that guided his life, as she embodied a true American spirit rooted in European values (see figure 2.1).[18]

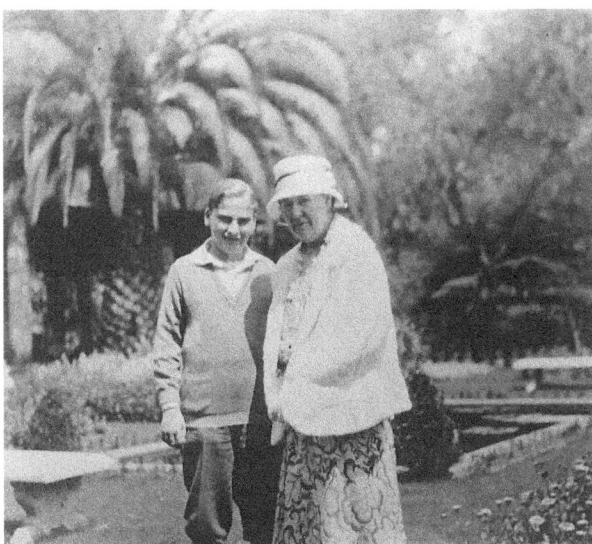

Figure 2.1. Menuhin and Willa Cather in Pasadena, 1931. Courtesy of the Foyle Menuhin Archive.

The family first met Cather in Paris in 1930, and the Menuhin children affectionately called her Aunt Willa.[19] In 1931 they reunited again in California when Yehudi was on his American tour and Cather received an honorary doctorate from the University of California. Menuhin bonded with her deeply as they took long walks together. He described her as "the most wholesome person I've ever known, crystal-pure and straightforward, never shrinking from saying things even if they hurt, so long as they were true things and were spoken with affection. She had the strength of the American soil which she loved so much and understood so well."[20] Aunt Willa was one of the few adults Marutha allowed to spend time alone with her children. In the insulated and even isolated Menuhin family, she was an intellectual and creative mother-figure to Menuhin, as opposed to his stern and perhaps overprotective real mother. When the family lived at the Ansonia Hotel in New York in 1932, the Menuhin children connected even more deeply with the great writer, who discussed literature, philosophy, and art with them as equals. She helped deepen their love of literature, and she presented the young violinist with poems by Heine and Goethe's *Faust*.[21] She even organized a Shakespeare club for the children, where they read plays together. Menuhin fondly recalls: "She was a rock one could always turn to, and I often did."[22]

Both Cather and Enesco penetrated the protective shield of the Menuhin family circle during Menuhin's early life, and their influences helped shape the violinist's curiosity and broaden his perspectives. Cather imparted culturally inclusive beliefs about humanity, while Enesco exposed him to Eastern European music and culture. Menuhin's experiences with both mentors help to explain why he felt drawn to pick up a book on yoga in 1951, and why he would embrace the yoga discipline for the rest of his life.

GROWING PAINS

Throughout his childhood and teenage years, Menuhin maintained an active schedule of concerts and rehearsals around the world. As he performed internationally with orchestras in major cities like Berlin, Paris, London, and New York, his status in the world of music grew rapidly. But beginning in March 1936, just before his twentieth birthday, Menuhin took an eighteen-month break from this nomadic life of concerts and rehearsals. Marutha had asked her son to give her a year before he "walks into the world a grown man."[23] This sabbatical would be an important time for Menuhin's intellectual and emotional maturation, as well as a time for him to explore the relationship of his body to his violin playing. The time off was filled with family outings and gatherings, as the Menuhins settled together in Los Gatos. Menuhin recalled how an "elegant gentleman from San Francisco, Mr. Keath, even taught us to dance the tango to 'Jealousy,'"[24] a tango by the Danish composer Jacob Gade, which Menuhin would record years later with the famous jazz violinist Stéphane Grappelli. The daughter of a Menuhin family friend from New York, Rosalie Leventritt, came to visit and sparked his first feelings of romance. When she left, Menuhin wrote a letter to Aunt Willa confiding his loss. She responded that "a little heartache is a good companion for a young man on his holiday," and she predicted that he would need the kind of wife much like his own mother who was "slight, heroic, delicate, unconquerable" with a more "disciplined nature than our [American] girls are likely to have."[25] Her letter would prove prophetic when Menuhin married his second wife, Diana Gould.

During his sabbatical from touring and rehearsals, Menuhin matured emotionally, intellectually, and musically. He began to contemplate a number of issues that would intersect with his future yoga practice, particularly a desire to develop a stronger sense of consciousness and knowledge about not only his music but also his body. By his own account, this maturation process was slow:

> Isolated in my day-to-day existence, as well as on the stage, I was slow in achieving a consciousness of life that comes comparatively early to most people, exposed as they are to contact in schools, at parties, athletic games, or work. The awakening, rebellion and readjustments that came to them naturally and gradually had passed me by. At the same time, my physical and intellectual growth were taking their normal course, eventually leading me to the realization that I must shift from my instinctive approach toward music to a conscious awareness and a readjustment, if need be.[26]

Menuhin understood that if he didn't make this transition then he "would be finished as an artist, sooner or later, in the way so many prodigies have failed when their instinct faltered."[27] Intellectually, Menuhin used this time off to study the repertory he had been playing from a more analytical perspective. He wanted to acquire knowledge of something he had previously only felt intuitively, and so he embarked on a quest to find "an organic relationship of parts towards each other and towards the whole."[28] Menuhin especially found such structural and expressive unity in Bach's six Sonatas and Partitas for Violin, in which he found "science, mysticism, and art are blended in a Holy Trinity."[29] As he revisited and analyzed these musical works, Menuhin felt that he "made a complete circle, returning to my original intuitive conception, but on a new level."[30] His understanding of music began to deepen as he realized that "the profundity of a mind may be measured by the extent to which it sees universal phenomena as part of a vast whole."[31] Such a quest for unity, which would occupy him for the rest of his life, resonates closely with his later devotion to yoga.

Throughout this period of intellectual maturation, Menuhin also began to search for knowledge and understanding about his physical body. He did not touch the violin for the first three months of his break. When he did finally pick it up again, he found a dramatic change. Gone was the effortless, intuitive connection between his instrument and sound that he had relied on for so long. Now, at age twenty-one, as he struggled to resume playing after the sabbatical, Menuhin encountered signs of physical problems and technical difficulties. He realized how little he really understood about the bodily mechanics of playing his instrument. Ysaÿe's admonitions about the importance of practicing scales and arpeggios turned out to be prescient. After this wake-up call, Menuhin recommitted himself to practicing, and he resolved to develop a stronger technical foundation and a deeper consciousness for playing the violin.

Menuhin began to perform again for audiences, first chamber music with friends at home, and then publicly in October 1937 with a recital in San Francisco. After that, he returned to the stage at the sold-out 4,450-seat San Francisco Memorial Opera House and garnered praise from critics as the "grown-up Yehudi, same rare spirit," whose performance was a "breath taking splash by the world's supreme violinist."[32] Menuhin then embarked on another concert tour in the States and abroad. He continued to meet with acclaim as he played in Seattle and Los Angeles, in Detroit for a CBS Music Hour radio concert with Hephzibah, and in New York under the baton of Enesco. His European stops traversed the British Isles, most notably at the Royal Albert Hall in London.

With a renewed energy for his music, Menuhin resumed seasonal concert tours with summer breaks. Over the coming years, his reputation on the world stage continued to grow, and he also began to contemplate his own maturation and passage out of youth into adulthood. By his own account, "Superficial appearance notwithstanding, I imagined that I had crossed the unmarked boundary that separates the men from the boys: I no longer had a teacher to spend summers with, I had progressed beyond regular tutelage, I was ready to fall in love. So I did."[33] Indeed, just before his twenty-second birthday, Menuhin met Nola Nicholas, a non-Jewish and high-society young woman from a wealthy Australian family, in 1938. Menuhin proposed soon after they met, and the two were wed a short two months later on May 26 in London.

The Coming Storm

The years between 1938, when Menuhin started touring again and married his first wife Nola Nicholas, and 1951, when he came across the little book on yoga in New Zealand, represent a difficult period in his life. During those thirteen years, Menuhin kept up a musical and personal drive that eventually wore out his mind and his body. As a world-famous Jewish violinist, he would confront some of the most challenging, exhausting, and traumatic situations of his life. Aside from the grueling demands of his concert career, Menuhin's new marriage plunged his personal and emotional life into turmoil. Like so many of his generation, his was a war marriage, but World War II itself would also shatter the world he thought he knew.

Although Menuhin and Nicholas had married with great fervor, the marriage didn't last. His parents wanted Menuhin and his sisters to marry young, perhaps to ensure an early transference to their own secure family life, and all the siblings complied. By Menuhin's own admission, the transition to adult life independent from the influence and authority of his parents was difficult. The couple lived for the first few months of their marriage with Menuhin's parents before moving into the guest cottage on the grounds of their home in Los Gatos.

As he returned to the international stage, Menuhin slowly took charge of his own concert schedule from his father—a process that pained Moshe as much as it empowered the young violinist. He continued his intensive world concert schedule in 1939, including his first tour of Latin America, before war broke out in Europe that fall. Nola gave birth to their first child, Menuhin's only daughter, Zamira, in September 1939. Their son Krov was born in August 1940 while Menuhin was on tour in Australia with Hephzibah. Menuhin later reflected idealistically that he "would have taught Nola of the innocence of Eden, she would have sponsored my assimilation in the world."[34] Yet, the young couple had strains on their marriage from the beginning, including from Menuhin's parents, who wanted them to live close by. While Nola accompanied Menuhin on his tours in the early months of their marriage, his busy concert schedule mostly left her home alone with the children.

War Years

With the declaration of war in September 1939, Europe was closed to Menuhin, and the world there as he knew it began its grim slide into catastrophe. When the United States entered the conflict in December 1941, Menuhin was exempted from the draft as the father of two children. He was not called up again until the last week of the war, and by waiting seven days to appear before the local draft board, he stayed out of the military.[35] Although spared from military duty, Menuhin threw himself into serving the war effort through music. Between 1942 and 1945, he gave hundreds of concerts for Allied troops and relief organizations, in addition to maintaining a regular concert schedule. With pianist Adolf Baller, he played for troops first in the Aleutian Islands and Hawaii, later in the Pacific Theater, and finally in Europe. Where civilian engagements took him, Menuhin offered additional concerts to the nearest army camp.[36] He was the first foreign concert artist to visit England in four years when he arrived there in 1943, and he sought ways to reach the people who were so battered by war. He performed with pianist Marcel Gazelle for British audiences in concert halls and factories, for the allied military forces, for US Army special services in their camps, and for charities; he even hid with people in shelters during German bombing raids.[37] Menuhin returned to Europe during the final two years of the war, traveling to the continent soon after the invasion of Normandy to give concerts in the liberated cities of Brussels, Antwerp, and Paris.

While doing his part for the war effort, Menuhin also matured into manhood. The harsh reality of war forced him to break out of the sheltered life he had been living since childhood: "More effectively than marriage, war cut me adrift from the past."[38] Playing for the military troops, rather than for cultured audiences in world-class concert halls, presented a new reality for Menuhin. Now he was playing for soldiers his own age in cafes and cabarets before or after they fought on the front lines. He had to adapt his performance routine in order to "woo his listeners."[39] "Before

I played for soldiers, music (though its purpose is communication) had fashioned round me a shell which I carried intact onto platforms and off again, in complicity with audiences who understood their part and mine in the operation. . . . Now I had to please men who had never attended a concert, who were not bred to its conventions, whose patience could not be relied upon, far less their informed appreciation."[40]

Menuhin found that in order to reach his audience of soldiers, he had to step beyond the impersonal barrier between classical performing artist and audience. He learned how to make conversation with the wounded in hospital wards and to remark upon the pieces he played: "Thus my [experience in the] war cracked open many inhibitions and helped me communicate with others, and thus my exclusive microcosm of music, violins and performance discovered its social dimension."[41] Even as he performed the "high-brow" classics of Bach, Beethoven, and Mendelssohn, Menuhin engaged with his listeners by connecting with their shared humanity. He felt the well-known and expressive "Ave Maria" by Schubert best calmed the troops. Where he had initially only hoped to bring pleasure and diversion, Menuhin was really "giving the men an escape back to the world of normal human emotions, of tenderness, romance, warmth, and also exaltation."[42] These lessons learned during the War about communication and reaching audiences bore fruit throughout his life as he shared his knowledge and understanding about music beyond the concert stage. Furthermore, they deepened the violinist's compassion for others, a foundational spiritual and yogic quality, and he found his involvement to be a "useful, humbling and finally exhilarating experience."[43]

As his relentless concert schedule during the war years took its toll, Menuhin himself reflected on how the emotional struggles in his personal life intersected with the technical challenges he was encountering. "Just as I had married without being prepared for marriage, so I played the violin without being prepared for violin playing, and it was inevitable that, the strain imposed by the breakdown in personal life coinciding with the unprecedented pressures of wartime touring, my lack of preparation would begin to tell."[44] Menuhin knew he had acquired bad habits from his intuitive, nonanalytical method of playing the violin, and although he had made efforts to address these issues earlier, the technical issues continued to trouble him. He realized that he would have to confront these problems so that he could recapture the natural ease that he felt was now "deserting" him.[45] In short, Menuhin had to become conscious as an adult of what he had always done unconsciously as a child.

Rather than cave in to these troubles, including lackluster reviews after off-nights, Menuhin's resilient nature persevered. With characteristic humility, courage, and open-mindedness, he began to search for solutions to his recurring technical difficulties—a pursuit that would occupy him for years to come and eventually bring him to yoga eight years later. Menuhin first realized that at the core of his problems with tension and fatigue was the mechanics of *motion*. He instinctively started to alter his practice routine by putting down the instrument and incorporating intervals of relaxation, deep breathing, and concentration on something other than the music at hand,[46] "brooding and groping" as he "reached his way to enlightenment."[47] He read classic violin technical books and consulted with other violin colleagues. Perhaps as a foreshadowing of his eventual turn to yoga to find answers, Menuhin also consulted with people outside the world of musical performance, experts in medicine, athletics, and gymnastics, including a tap dancer and a runner.

As the war years continued to grind on, Menuhin experienced a significant personal and professional transformation. In November 1943 in New York, Menuhin met Béla Bartók, an encounter that Menuhin would describe, despite the tragic context, as one of the most profound of his life. The great Hungarian composer was, according to Menuhin, "just another refugee, swept by the tide of war onto American shores, living in a modest apartment in New York City, ill, poor and known outside of Hungary to only a happy few."[48] Like his fascination with Enesco and gypsy music, Menuhin loved how Bartók's music had an exotic, or what he referred to as "Eastern," aura. In keeping with his own understanding of "unity in diversity" and universal truths, he admired how Bartók "elevated folk music to universal validity, so he gave noble dimensions to human emotions."[49] Menuhin commissioned the composer to write a solo sonata for him, which the violinist premiered at Carnegie Hall in November 1944, less than a year before Bartók died. Menuhin cited the performance as one of the great milestones of his life.

While the strain of maintaining a rigorous concert schedule made a normal family life nearly impossible, Menuhin's extended absences from home were only one contributing factor to the end of his first marriage. Owing to his extremely protected childhood, Menuhin was ill-equipped to deal with relationships when he and Nola rushed into marriage. They barely knew each other, they were both very young, and they had very different temperaments and interests. By 1944 the couple realized they were "hopelessly at odds." [50] Although they did not divorce immediately, they separated that year and continued to struggle through the marriage for three more painful years, which Menuhin would later describe as "the most troubled and mismanaged" of his life.[51] Years later in a letter, Menuhin's sister Hephzibah, whose first marriage suffered the same painful end, identifies the essence of their relationship struggles as rooted in their upbringing. She describes how, although their education at home provided the means to achieve mastery of music, their sheltered life rendered them useless to solve everyday problems. "As soon as our structure became invaded by the utterly different values of other people, we were helpless in coping with the conflict it set up between what we had been taught, and what we were being taught."[52]

In September 1944, while traversing the Atlantic on tours between the United States and England, Menuhin, now twenty-eight years old, met Diana Gould, who was three and a half years his senior. Although Menuhin immediately felt that Diana was meant for him, his marriage to Nola had not yet ended, and he would later describe the next two years as the worst period of his life.[53] With London as his base from 1945 to 1947, Menuhin would see Diana when he was in town. As a trained dancer, Diana was a woman of discipline, artistry, and wit, and she matched the musician's temperament. In those visits, they attended concerts and got to know each other as kindred spirits in the arts, and Menuhin's "sadness fell away."[54] Diana remembers how, as he slowly opened up to her, she "sensed that he was as shocked and sad as a child who has misunderstood something of great value and importance, and who cannot find the way out."[55] As he was still tied to Nola and his children in California, Menuhin struggled to accept that his marriage was ending.

Riddled with indecision and uncertainty, Menuhin lacked focus. He withdrew from family and friends into an isolated space where even his dear sister Hephzibah and beloved Aunt Willa could not reach him. Unaccustomed to taking care of himself, he gained weight and "was pale and flabby, moving about like the tired man he was."[56] Menuhin reflects on this dark period, feeling remorseful about his inability to take action as he struggled to realign his beliefs and values:

> Some mistakes one makes are fruitful; one gains strength and wisdom by them; but this one I deeply regret, for nothing was gained by it and Diana, who asked nothing, was subjected to many months of agonizing uncertainty, committed to me yet never knowing when I might reappear or for how long.

How far I had fallen from my childhood dream of universal peace and harmony! How helpless music proved to be in this personal defeat! I had estranged myself from parents, wife, even children.[57]

In the end, Nola initiated divorce proceedings in 1947. Finally released from the inertia of ambivalence, Menuhin married Diana in London on October 19, 1947. For the rest of his life, she provided a continuous source of love and support to Menuhin's life and work. He, in turn, practically worshiped her, even as he allowed her to manage his life. Together they had two sons: Gerard, born in 1948, and Jeremy, born in 1951. Sadly, they lost their newborn third son Alexis in 1955.

Humanitarian Service and Reconciliation

In July 1945, just three months after the war ended and despite a grueling concert and touring schedule, Menuhin returned to Germany. He felt driven to be of service to the world through music, now as a healing force. Compelled to witness for himself the horrors of the Nazi concentration camps and "to offer the living victims the sorrow, the repentance, the solidarity of the unharmed," he gave a concert with composer/pianist Benjamin Britten in Bergen-Belsen to raise funds for "displaced persons."[58] This drive to help after the war would remain strong, and Menuhin traveled throughout liberated Europe in 1945 to give other concerts. He visited Prague in October and Moscow in November, where he also met the legendary violinist David Oistrakh (with whom he would maintain a friendship until his death in 1974). Menuhin's parents had emigrated to the United States from Russia, and now, at the source of his own heritage, the violinist connected with the "language, the rhythms, the landscape" of his ancestors in Russia and into his "mother's real and dream worlds."[59] Just as Menuhin had discovered the music and spirit of Romania through Enesco, his visit to Russia inspired "yet profounder depths to that strangely familiar homeland called the East."[60] The same connection to the East would resonate with him again in India seven years later.

Menuhin continued his intense concert schedule in 1946. In May he toured Romania, where he reunited with Enesco after not seeing him since 1939 in Paris. Giving daily concerts for nearly two weeks with his beloved mentor, Menuhin received an extraordinary welcome from Romanians.

They greeted him as a disciple of their country's great composer, Enesco; as an American, the country that stood for generosity and liberation after the war; and as a Jew, since Bucharest had become the Jewish capital of Europe after offering refuge to thousands who had escaped persecution.[61] Their concerts raised a fair amount of money, which Menuhin and Enesco gave to the Red Cross, Jewish charities, and young Romanian musicians.[62]

Menuhin also visited Hungary in 1946. He was welcomed as a champion of Bartók's music, and he played the sonata that the great composer had written for him. While in Hungary, Menuhin deepened his understanding of East/West cross-fertilizations. He observed how the country, and the former Austro-Hungarian empire in general, drew on a mix of cultures, including Hungarian, Turkish, Balkan, German, French, Italian, and Jewish traditions.[63] Menuhin also met Hungary's other renowned composer, Zoltán Kodály. Before he left the country, Menuhin tried to commission a work by him, but it was never completed.[64]

It was one thing for Menuhin to perform in liberated countries after the war, but it was entirely another thing to play in the country that instigated the horror—Germany. With his characteristic openness, and in this case idealistic innocence, Menuhin played in Berlin in 1946 and again in 1947 at the invitation of the American military government. He wanted to go "as a Jew who might keep alive the German guilt and repentance, and as a musician offering something to live for."[65] His humanistic conviction to convey "something of the essential brotherhood of man" had a practical goal as well—to raise money for the Jewish community, the Berlin Academy of Music, the Berlin Philharmonic, and the Free University.[66] Menuhin performed with legendary conductor of the Berlin Philharmonic Wilhelm Furtwängler (1886–1954), who had stayed in Germany during the war. This stoked a great deal of controversy. Although Furtwängler never joined the Nazi party or supported Hitler, and in fact helped many Jewish musicians escape the country, he was nonetheless criticized for staying at all. In turn, Menuhin was criticized for performing for Germans and with Fürtwangler. Yet Menuhin stood by his idealistic principles and sided with those of the great conductor—that the power of music should transcend politics. Menuhin believed that Fürtwangler's reasons for staying in Germany deserved compassion, given that the conductor's "musical vision could best be made to exist in Germany, by a German orchestra before a German public."[67]

Menuhin's commitment to using music to reach all people after the war in Germany would bring with it still more controversy. In 1947, he asked the American authorities in Berlin to organize a recital for him at a camp where displaced people, mostly Jews, were still living. It took place at a cinema in the suburbs of the Deuppel Center, one of many such camps that still existed two years after the war, and where many traumatized survivors of the Nazi camps remained. Despite Menuhin's noble intentions, fewer than fifty displaced persons attended,[68] although the cinema could seat more than a thousand people. Menuhin played for the sparse audience, learning afterward that someone had organized a boycott because Menuhin had played for "murderers of the Jewish people, the Germans."[69] Menuhin resolved to face this conflict head-on, and the next day he went to the camp to meet the organizer and the people. He recalls:

> When we reached the wire fences and guard gates of the Deuppel Centre, it was to feel with the keenness of personal experience how slow was its inmates' return from the tomb. . . . Two military policeman escorted us into the hut and, with some difficulty, pushed us through the dense crowd inside to the stage. Boos, hisses, and imprecations followed us all the way. Since the noise showed no signs of abating, I stood up to confront my judges . . . "I cannot blame anyone for this bitterness . . . you have suffered too much. And still I do say that you cannot rebuild your life on your suffering. Don't let it be said that we have only learned the worst of our enemies! We Jews don't beg; we work! We are the best cobblers, the best tailors, the best doctors, the best musicians. That's what it means to be a Jew! I have come to Germany to restore that image, to show how false was Hitler's caricature. That's why I'm here."[70]

After such a grim confrontation, his words moved the people to friendliness and forgiveness, and they appealed for a second concert. Sadly, Menuhin could not comply since he was leaving Berlin the next day. That evening, the organizer of the boycott came to the musician and apologized for his accusations, saying that "had another concert been given, everyone would have gone."[71] The organizer later told an American reporter, "Perhaps it is too much to expect that those who have not experienced persecution and camps should understand our feelings."[72] Yet, Menuhin *could* understand this man's hatred of his oppressor, even as he could sympathize with Furtwängler's reasons for staying in Germany during the War. As his worldview had enough depth to embrace both sides of a conflict, Menuhin believed desire for vengeance alone, excluding all other responses, was a weakness.[73] His approach to compassion always called for reconciliation.

Although Menuhin had made peace with the people at the Deuppel Center, he subsequently faced other boycotts by Jews in both North and South America.[74] Still, the hardest test to come after the War was his tour in Israel. With his sister Hephzibah at the piano and Diana at his side, Menuhin went to the newly formed country even in the face of death threats. "The gauntlet of universal peace thrown down," he made a whirl-wind tour, giving two recitals a day over the course of twelve days.[75] While in Israel, he also connected to his ancestry, since this was the country where his parents had first met as refugees from Russia. Menuhin later described gaining a better understanding of his father's legacy when he visited a college in Jerusalem similar to the one his father had attended and imagined him "wearing long side curls, walking the narrow streets shoulder to shoulder with his Arab friends, fellows in common disapproval of the Turkish overlord."[76] Although Moshe had abandoned Zionism, he continued to champion the cause of the weaker against the more powerful, a trait that Menuhin clearly inherited from his father. During the trip, Menuhin also met the president of the new country, Chaim Weizmann, and his wife. He subsequently invited them to Gstaad, Switzerland, where the Menuhins would build a house in the late 1950s.[77]

In South America, Menuhin toured Argentina—where the Jews of Buenos Aires welcomed instead of boycotted him—as well as Brazil, Peru, Ecuador, and Venezuela. He found Peru fascinating and made the pilgrimage to Machu Picchu in 1949 by foot—"the severest physical test I have ever undergone."[78] Menuhin also performed in North Africa in 1951. His tour of South Africa in 1950, where he first encountered apartheid, presented a special challenge. To reach all the people of the country, Menuhin maneuvered his way to perform duplicate concerts for black audiences on the mornings of his regular evening concerts, which only whites could attend.[79] He returned to this racially divided country in 1956. After that, however, Menuhin's conscience did not allow him to play there again, and he returned to South Africa only when apartheid ended in 1995.

By 1951, the year he discovered yoga, Menuhin found himself at a low point in his life, standing at a crossroads of physical, emotional, and probably spiritual forces. Despite the new stability and happiness that he found in his second marriage to Diana, the failure of his first marriage was still an emotional weight. He was now a middle-aged man whose rigorous self-imposed concert schedule had propelled him to perform nonstop for nearly fifteen years, as he pushed himself to celebrate life through music in the midst of a traumatic war and a bitter peace. The demands of his concert schedule left little time to recover, emotionally or physically, from the exhaustion of war. His physical struggles with the violin continued too and even intensified as his body aged and his agility lessened. Menuhin was actively seeking a remedy that would allow him to develop another way of playing the violin—one that would permit him to still embrace his instincts but with a stronger understanding of the body's mechanisms. Once he established the direction of this search, every experience pushed him toward this consciousness, including his "own practice, exchanges with other violinists, the laws of physics, a passage to India, and of course specifically yoga, which taught [him] lessons it would have taken years to elaborate for [him]self."[80] Menuhin beautifully summarizes his experience of how yoga "first and foremost . . . made its contribution to my quest to understand consciously the mechanics of violin playing, a quest which by 1951, had long been one of the themes of my life."[81]

Menuhin's encounter with yoga in 1951 and subsequent disciple-guru connection with B. K. S. Iyengar presented the timely solution to solving his problems. While yoga directed Menuhin's violin quest as it trained his body to acquire strength, balance, economy of energy, unity of motion, and release of tension, it also provided a framework for a more holistic approach to life. As Menuhin embraced his yoga practice, he began to consciously balance care of the physical body through exercise, sleep, and proper diet with mental and spiritual preparation. He sought to maintain a fit spiritual condition, as "the state of mind, the state of nerve, the state of heart are as important as the state of muscle."[82] Furthermore, as Menuhin embarked on his mission to understand the mechanics of violin playing, his guru Iyengar's methodical approach to yoga resonated with his quest. By 1954, Menuhin considered Iyengar to be his "best violin teacher," as the engraving he put on the Omega watch given to Iyengar that September in Gstaad testified.

Chapter 3

Yoga Path of Action

Menuhin's Musical Performances and Yoga Advocacy

The first ten years of Menuhin's engagement with yoga demonstrate his remarkable commitment and enthusiasm for a practice that had largely been unknown not only to him but also to Europe and the United States. Between 1952 and 1962, as he integrated yoga into his daily life and nurtured his close relationship with Iyengar, Menuhin's life trajectory also shifted. During those ten years, he broadened his musical activities beyond performing solely as a concert violinist. Following his guru's body/mind/spirit conception of yoga, Menuhin's life demonstrated a consistent and notable embrace of yogic principles in the physical realm, or the dimension of the body, in the years after he began working with Iyengar. While Menuhin's physical yoga practice of *asana* and *pranayama* provided him with a way to maintain a healthy body and mind, it was just one part of a larger embrace of yogic ideas and principles in his musical practice. Menuhin's own physical yoga practice not only improved his violin technique and helped him sustain a fast-paced and high-profile performance schedule, but the discipline's deeper philosophical and spiritual values must have also influenced how his professional activities branched out into new directions.

In this chapter, I will examine how Menuhin expanded his work as a classical violinist to become a conductor, an impresario, and a performer of world music. He sought to effect meaningful change in the world through music as he forged a close connection with Iyengar and absorbed an understanding of yoga. Menuhin also became an advocate for his guru's teachings in Europe by sharing his newfound practice with colleagues and family. And, as Menuhin became enamored of Indian culture and music, especially the art of improvisation, through his yoga practice he transferred this fascination with all things Indian to his work as a performer and festival organizer. In turn, Menuhin's work related to Indian music and spirituality exerted a broader cultural influence in the 1960s, both in the classical and popular music realms.

Menuhin's new activities, including organization of festivals, advocacy of Iyengar, and promotion of world music, can be understood as embodying the pathway of *karmayoga*, or the Yoga of Action. Following this pathway, a yogi exerts the necessary effort, or the burning zeal of *tapas*, in the world to do, make, and accomplish things according to their *dharma*[1] yet practice nonattachment to the results of their actions. Viewing Menuhin's life through the lens of the Yoga of Action demonstrates these yoga principles at work.

Menuhin humbly exhibited a non-egocentric attitude in his musical work by using music as a means to promote the spirit of unity to his audiences—an idea that reached all the way back to his childhood. The motivating fire behind his performances and other music projects was not fueled by a desire for self-promotion. Rather, Menuhin's musical work reflected important yogic principles, set forth by Iyengar, to dedicate the fruits of one's actions to the greater good of humanity. His ethics embodied both the *yamas* and *niyamas*, those universal and individual codes of conduct and attitudes that fortify the yoga practitioner and reinforce how discipline and practice pave the way to freedom.

Renewed Performer and Conductor of Classical Music

Like the *klesas* that present obstacles to liberation for the yogi, Menuhin was well aware of impediments that could block his violin playing, which he himself identified as "physical, mental, emotional," and how mechanical playing could take over "without full participation of heart and mind."[2] To stay fit in body, mind, and spirit, Menuhin established a regular yoga practice that was as much a part of his daily routine as practicing the violin. Taking care of his body was paramount. While he adhered to the yogic belief that we are *not* the body, he felt it was his responsibility to continually improve his violin technique in order to ensure its precision and fluidity as the vehicle for his musical expression. He described his morning ritual as rising at seven o'clock, bathing, and doing his exercises. He varied his favorite yoga postures to include "slow and fast, heavy and light, inverted body postures, hanging by the arms and by the legs—all the variations I can think of."[3] Then, after a wholesome breakfast (he loved porridge), he would commence to practice the violin. On concert days, he would do some more exercises to limber up his body and again practice the violin before the performance.

As a working musician who spent much of his time in hotel rooms, Menuhin found yoga *asana* and *pranayama* to be well-suited to his concert-tour lifestyle, and he was enthusiastically open about his newfound yoga practice. During Menuhin's initial trip to India in 1952 to support the Famine Relief Fund, the *Times of India* highlighted the great violinist's interest in yoga. Upon his return, the press grabbed on to the novelty, and Menuhin began making headlines in the States. As he continued his rigorous concert schedule, including his annual American tour, the press found renewed expression in his playing and highlighted his fascination with yoga. Following Menuhin's twenty-fifth-anniversary New York recital debut performance in January 1953, the *New York Times* music critic Howard Taubman also pointed out Menuhin's improved artistry and technique in his review:

> The Yehudi Menuhin who played in Carnegie Hall last night performed like an important new violinist. The importance lay in the thrust and personality Mr. Menuhin revealed as an interpreter. It was as though he had moved up to a higher level of accomplishment, a level one had expected him to achieve sooner. But maturity as an artist is not won easily. . . . In recent years there has been evidence of a struggle going on within him. Whatever private difficulties he has had with his art, he seemed to have conquered them.[4]

A few days later, an article in *Life Magazine* confirmed Taubman's assessment as it described Menuhin's "revitalized" appearance in a New York recital following recent "disappointing" performances that "stirred critics to superlatives unmatched since the violinist made his blazing debut at the age of 8. . . . Menuhin, now 36, is serious about yoga, ranks it and sleep as more important even than violin practice."[5] The article features photos of Menuhin with his first yoga teacher Vithalda practicing *sim-hasana* (Lion Pose), *pindasana* (Embryo Pose), and *ardha matsyendrasana* (Half Lord of the Fishes Pose); the technique *neti kriya* (nasal cleansing); and *pranayama*.

During Menuhin's second trip to India in 1954, the press highlighted his interest in yoga while writing rave reviews of his classical violin performances. Menuhin made a big splash throughout his six-week tour in Bombay, Delhi, Calcutta, and Madras, and the stellar reviews from the Indian press also drew attention to his interest in Indian music with such headlines as "Menuhin—The Artist and The Yogi."[6] Back in the West during the 1954–1955 season, Menuhin again caught the attention of the press with his yoga practice and studies with Iyengar. Headlines like "Yoga Turns Yehudi Upside Down" in the *Arkansas Gazette*, "Yehudi Stands on His Head" in *People Today*, and "Yehudi Is a Yogi" in the *Montreal Canada Star* documented sessions between guru and disciple in India and Gstaad.[7] The *Weekend Magazine* of the *Montreal Canada Star* summed up Menuhin's yoga-music connection: "As he has striven for perfection as a musician, so he strives for a flawless performance in the demanding techniques of yoga."[8]

The press also found humor in how Menuhin demonstrated yoga poses while on his concert tours. He even shared his practice with heads of state like David Ben-Gurion in Israel. Menuhin met him several times, once in the concert hall in the Golan Heights, where the Israeli Philharmonic Orchestra performed. Menuhin recalled: "Ben-Gurion was the second statesman in whose company I stood on my head, for he too practiced yoga."[9] A newspaper cartoon clipping depicted the occasion with an apt definition of yoga from the Concise Oxford Dictionary: "YOGA: Hindu system of philosophic meditation and asceticism designed to effect the reunion of the devotee's soul with the universal spirit."[10]

In the late 1950s Menuhin began to diversify his performing activities to include conducting. He expanded his professional musical work by collaborating with fellow musicians in chamber orchestras and ensembles, reflecting another way his life followed the path of the Yoga of Action. Menuhin's first conducting experience dates from 1958, when he fulfilled the standard role of the concert master/conductor of the baroque chamber orchestra for his EMI recording of the Bach Brandenburg Concertos.[11] As he took on more orchestral activities in the 1960s and 70s, Menuhin also carried his physical yoga practice with him. He even demonstrated how he could stand on his head while dressed in concert attire.

Music Impresario

Along with his own performances, Menuhin's extensive efforts to develop, organize, and participate in major musical festivals across Europe further reflect his engagements with the principles of *karmayoga*. As Europe recovered from the trauma of World War II and a number of summer music festivals began to spring up around the continent and Great Britain, Menuhin became an ambassador for music. He appeared at one of the early ones, the Aldeburgh Festival in Suffolk, "where in the midst of the post-war austerities, Benjamin Britten found a way of playing his own music and other peoples' with his friends."[12] The two were still connected through the bond they had built on their joint tour of the horrifying concentration camps after the war, and Menuhin supported Britten by performing at the festival just for the love of "meeting colleagues and making music with them."[13]

Menuhin's involvement and influence in various music organizations and festivals, including the Gstaad, Bath, and the Commonwealth Arts Festivals, also provided him with venues to regularly bring Iyengar to Europe. Through Menuhin's endorsement, Iyengar was able to bring yoga to other musicians and colleagues in the violinist's circle, including the well-known pianist Clifford Curzon and the rising-star cellist Jacqueline du Pré in London.[14] Menuhin also introduced Iyengar to European dig-nitaries and royalty, including Elisabeth of Bavaria, the Queen Mother of Belgium (1876–1965), herself a violinist and patron of music who was then in her eighties. Iyengar taught her on numerous trips until just a few months before she died.

The Gstaad Festival

In his extensive involvement as the organizer of other summer festivals, Menuhin exemplified the yoga quality of *sattva* (equanimity), even as he was driven by the burning zeal of *tapas* to perform. His famous Gstaad Festival in Switzerland offers the best example of his goodwill as his embrace of yoga intersected with his festival work. Over the course of thirty-nine years, the Gstaad Festival carried the stamp of Menuhin's humble and idealistic personality as it became a center for music and yoga (see figure 3.1).

The Gstaad Festival started in 1957 as a summer gathering of Menuhin and his musician friends, including Benjamin Britten and his partner

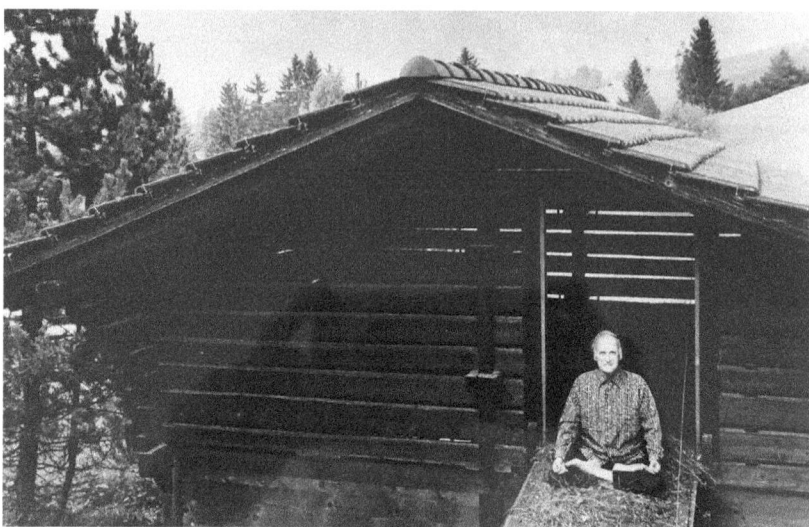

Figure 3.1. Menuhin in *padmasana* (Lotus Pose) in Gstaad, undated but probably from the mid-1980s. Courtesy of Foyle Menuhin Archive.

tenor Peter Pears, to offer intimate chamber performances at the church in the nearby town of Saanen. By July 1960, when Menuhin established a more permanent base in Gstaad by building his own summer home there, the festival had already begun to expand. By the 1980s, it had evolved into a full-fledged professional festival that included semi-staged operas and symphonic works under a large performance tent. Menuhin ran the Gstaad Festival until 1996, when he gave his final public violin performance there. He then passed the director's baton to the violinist and conductor Gidon Kremer, who stayed in the position for two years. Eventually the post was offered to Eleanor Hope and renamed "Menuhin Festival Gstaad."[15] Now called the Gstaad Menuhin Festival and Academy, it is still flourishing today.[16]

Even before the festival officially began in 1957, Menuhin's yoga practice with Iyengar influenced both his family and his close musical colleagues in Gstaad. Diana Menuhin recalls the guru's arrival there that first summer in 1954 while looking out the window during breakfast:

Up the drive, his soaking *dhoti* [a long loincloth traditionally worn by Hindu men in southern Asia] clinging to his muscular legs, strode Mr. B. Y. [*sic*] S. Iyengar, Guru-in-Chief to

Yehudi Menuhin. With a muffled sound, Y scuttled from the table and shot into the hall to open the front door and give Mr. Iyengar a welcoming hug. I stood while the puddle round poor Iyengar gradually reached his ankles and waited. "Darling, didn't I tell you?" Y asked innocently. Mr. Iyengar is spending the summer with us.[17]

Menuhin envisioned yoga sessions in Gstaad to be a "communal activity," where the entire family would gather at seven in the morning for the day's exercises.[18] Menuhin's sphere of yoga influence spread beyond his family at Gstaad. As Menuhin regularly invited Iyengar to return to Switzerland in the 1950s and 1960s, a number of other musicians and staff who participated in the festival also became fervent disciples of Iyengar's, including the pianists Curzon and Lili Kraus and the secretary of the Asian Music Circle, Angela Marris.

FESTIVALS IN THE UNITED KINGDOM

Menuhin's extensive organizing and development of other festivals in his adult life underscores his commitment to important areas of yogic practice, especially as related to the concepts of unity and diversity that he first learned as a child from Willa Cather. While the Gstaad Festival in Switzerland was his own creation, Menuhin helped run others in the UK, including the Bath Festival from 1959 to 1968, the Commonwealth Arts Festival in 1965, and the Windsor Festival from 1969 to 1972. Over the course of thirteen years while serving as the artistic director of the Bath Festival and joint artistic director of the Windsor Festival, Menuhin put his personal artistic stamp on music programming that reflected his own "history, preferences, and aspirations."[19] In keeping with his broad multicultural perspective and worldview, Menuhin built bridges between performers and audiences to increase global understanding and harmony through music, expanding the programs at the Bath Festival to embrace world music and jazz. Menuhin's programs reached across location and period to highlight the artistry of musicians from India, Iran, Greece, and Russia. Ever the cultural adventurer, Menuhin also created a "musical encounter" in the 1963 festival, where he and John Dankworth, along with other assorted jazz and classical musicians, improvised in a performance of William Russo's *Music for Violin and Jazz Orchestra* conducted by Raymond Leppard.[20]

Menuhin also had the opportunity to put his yoga-influenced ideals into action in the fall of 1965, when he was invited to collaborate in the one-time-only Commonwealth Arts Festival, which sponsored concerts and events in several British cities including London, Liverpool, Cardiff, and Glasgow. As one of the organizers, Menuhin got to observe and hear firsthand the Indian and African musicians who participated in the festival.[21] His musical knowledge and understanding expanded from such exposure to world music, and he gained new insights into the deeper connections between music and culture. In the element of rhythm in Indian and African music, for example, he realized how the former relies on an individual player and the latter on the collective group, enabling him to see "a first close view of the music of yet another culture which added perspective to the links between social and musical organization."[22]

Iyengar's Advocate in the West

Menuhin also embodied the Yoga of Action by advocating for Iyengar in the West, and the clarity and accessibility of Iyengar Yoga began to take root. With their guru-student relationship firmly established in trust, and their friendship cemented with mutual respect and admiration, Iyengar and Menuhin began to forge a professional relationship as colleagues. As this new level of their relationship became woven into Menuhin's musical network and projects, it became mutually beneficial and influential. Iyengar provided expert yoga instruction to Menuhin and his circle, while the violinist promoted Iyengar's yoga demonstrations and classes. Iyengar recounts: "My contact with Menuhin was prestigious to us both. Members of the public started to appreciate my work. I reiterate that the happy turn of events was entirely due to the grace of God."[23]

BUILDING A REPUTATION AND FOLLOWING

When Iyengar came to Gstaad for the first time in the summer of 1954, Menuhin also brought him as a guest to London, where he had a home, to teach yoga. While yoga had started to appear on people's radar in the UK as a health and fitness practice through such channels as Theos Bernard's book *Hatha Yoga* (1950), Desmond Dunn's book *Yoga for Everyman* (1951), and articles in the magazine *Health & Strength*,[24] it would be another decade before yoga took off through the adult education classes of local education authorities in the UK.[25] In this first visit, Iyengar started to build a London following with only two students, Menuhin and the Polish pianist Witold Malcużyński. Zamira recalls: "I was present at an evening of demonstrations by Mr. Iyengar that my father arranged with Mrs. Pandit, [Prime Minister] Nehru's sister, at the Indian High Commission in London. This attracted a lot of interest, as yoga and Indian music were until then familiar to a select few in the West."[26]

As Iyengar returned annually to the city to teach yoga, the number of private classes for Menuhin's musician and non-musician friends grew year by year.[27] As a result, Iyengar Yoga began to grow there as the guru moved from private to public classes. Even as the word about Iyengar spread, it would still take seven years and hundreds of demonstrations to establish his reputation and attract enough people to give his first official class in 1961.[28]

Iyengar's classes in London coincided with other types of yoga being taught in the UK during this period, such as Pranayama Yoga (Sunita Cabral, 1932–1970) and the Wheel of British Yoga (Wilfred Clark, 1898– 1981). However, Iyengar Yoga would become the most well-established and organized type of yoga in the UK in the 1960s, largely through its endorsement from the Inner London Education Authority, Iyengar's own systematic "bureaucratic framework" of training his students to transmit his approach in his absence,[29] and Iyengar's book *Light on Yoga*. Iyengar's physically challenging classes focused on *asana* and *pranayama*, ending with a period of complete relaxation.[30]

Iyengar credits "the healing aspects of yoga," especially as he practiced it with ailing people, as the catalyst for yoga finally catching on in the West.[31] Iyengar wanted to make the science of yoga accessible to people. He taught in a practical way that focused on alignment of the body while still holding to his larger mission to teach people to apply their mind and intelligence while practicing the discipline.[32] Still, Iyengar's means to teach and disseminate yoga through performances and demonstrations, including staged venues, reached Westerners as well. As yoga scholar Suzanne Newcombe writes:

> When B. K. S. Iyengar came to Britain to promote yoga in the 1960s, he attempted to make use of every platform he could in order to inspire interest in the subject. His stages included the living rooms of the elite in Highgate [e.g., Menuhin and his circle], the Everyman's Theater in Hampstead, the stage offered

by BBC television broadcasting, the large stage of London's
Quaker Meeting Hall in Euston, and a sell-out demonstration
at the Barbican in London (a major classical music venue) in
1984.[33]

Iyengar himself recalled how he was "when occasion demanded, a
performer and an artist."[34] With his strong stage presence that included
"qualities of precision, skillfulness, and artistry,"[35] he surely paralleled
the charisma of Menuhin as a performer. As both were masters of their
respective crafts, and had already established a soul connection early in
their relationship, they shared yet another similarity and point of connection in their artistic performances on stage.

Menuhin personally helped arrange Iyengar's trips to Europe during
the 1950s and early 1960s. While he always benefitted from his work
with Iyengar, Menuhin also valued Iyengar's presence on the world stage
as a great artist/teacher who transcended boundaries of race and culture.
By the late 1950s Menuhin was not only introducing his guru into the
international arena, but he was also advocating for cultural inclusiveness
and challenging prejudice in the arts. Such activities demonstrate how
Menuhin's life embodied yoga beyond just the physical practice of *asana*
by implementing strong moral principles in keeping with the Yoga of
Action. For example, he introduced the International Arts League of Youth
in South Africa to Iyengar in hopes of encouraging them to break their
color bar. As a Jew, Menuhin firmly believed "any international organization must of course include different races," and he could not "accept the
privileges for one race while permitting the exemption of other races."[36]

Menuhin sent a copy of this letter to Iyengar, which is also in the
Ramamani Iyengar Memorial Yoga Institute (RIMYI) Archive. An undated
"Message from Yehudi Menuhin" followed this letter, most likely written
to introduce one of Iyengar's demonstrations in either London or Gstaad.
It illustrates how Menuhin promoted his guru as an artist and how he
took great care to explain the true practice of yoga to an audience before
Iyengar performed:

> This evening you are going to see a man who is as dedicated
> to his art as any musician or painter. His is an art reduced to
> the very simplest in a sense, yet one of the most complicated
> because it requires no instrument at all. It requires only the
> instrument you are born with—your body. . . . To perfect this

art requires a lifetime of patient and persistent effort, always trying to perfect this instrument we have been given. . . .

Mr. Iyengar will show you all kinds of postures—called *asanas*—which have been developed over thousands of years . . . by people who sought concentration, who sought balance of life. . . . This discipline of yoga was developed in order to enable people to free their mind and body from any irrelevant external and disturbing factors so that they would not have any distraction.

I do hope this evening will leave you with a better understanding of what is implied by the word Yoga as well as a sense of wonder at the precision, refinement and beauty of Mr. Iyengar's art. He demonstrates to perfection how a man can raise himself to his own highest potential by the practice of yoga. May this performance be an inspiration to many to follow in his footsteps.[37]

Menuhin's own words capture how deeply he was engaged with yoga and what he understood the discipline to be. While he valued and understood the dedicated practice needed to master *asana*, he understood yoga to be more than simply achieving the precision of physical exercise. He had absorbed Iyengar's own view of how yoga was a means to quiet the mind, to strengthen concentration, and to attain balance in life.

Menuhin organized lectures, classes, and demonstrations for Iyengar through numerous channels in England. The two men stayed connected through their letters, where Menuhin typically proposed plans, reported on the status of his yoga practice, and conveyed family news and greetings. He wrote early in 1960 shortly after he had moved to Highgate Village in London: "I think about you very often, in fact hardly a day would pass without a letter of mine, would I write each time I thought of you, which is at least each time I stand on my head or do one of the other exercises."[38] Menuhin also commented how happy he was to learn that Iyengar's eldest daughter was "following in his footsteps."[39]

Menuhin's career was thriving in the late 1950s and early 1960s as he maintained his robust international performance schedule and became an active festival organizer and educator. In addition to his work with the Gstaad Festival and the Bath Festival in 1959, he was eager to bring Iyengar to London to perform and lecture in 1960. He had been work-ing with the Asian Music Circle in London and hoped it would soon be financially stable enough to help bring Iyengar to the city. Menuhin intended to secure a TV appearance on the BBC and other engagements for Iyengar, although the BBC appearance didn't actually happen until three years later. He continued to involve the Queen Mother in Brussels in Iyengar's visits, and he enlisted the help of other musicians in his circle studying yoga with Iyengar, like Lili Kraus, to help with the arrangements.

Iyengar did indeed come to Europe in the summer of 1960 to teach yoga, and his first stop was with Menuhin in London. Iyengar reflected on working with the entire family, where even Menuhin's mother joined the yoga classes: "Ma [the nickname for Menuhin's mother] & Jeremy must be as active in the morning as they were when I was working with them. I am really so happy that they could learn so much in so short a time . . . I am sure you are also maintaining as you did yesterday. I pray God to bless you forever with everything. That is all I can do for you. With deepest affections, B. K. S. Iyengar."[40]

Next Iyengar went to Brussels to teach the Queen Mother. Apparently, she enjoyed doing headstand as much as Menuhin did, as Iyengar reported to Menuhin after he saw her the morning he arrived: "She looks the same accept [sic] she has the hay fever. She asked me whether she could stand on her head again. I said that I would try [to help her]."[41] Now both Menuhin and his guru enjoyed a personal relationship with the Queen Mother as they connected through yoga. Iyengar further consolidated their plan for Menuhin to come to Brussels, saying the Queen told him he should bring his daughter and stay at the chateau rather than a hotel.

With Menuhin's help, Iyengar was beginning to develop his own network in Europe, expanding his teaching practice and, consequently, bringing yoga to a part of the world where it had existed only minimally before. Rather than Menuhin initiating all the arrangements for his guru, Iyengar was the one making plans for his visit to Switzerland that summer of 1960. Among his new students were some of the most high-profile personalities in Europe. He had already been in touch with the Indian ambassador in Berne to arrange for his demonstrations in early September and also to invite the Swiss president.[42] While still in Brussels, Iyengar wrote again to Menuhin to say the Queen was looking forward to his visit and how "she is keeping up fine health & enjoys yoga enormously," and he commended Menuhin, saying, "I am personally indebted to you and am again looking forward for our meeting. I am so happy that you are doing yoga regularly."[43]

With yoga now deeply entrenched in his daily life, Menuhin stayed in close touch with Iyengar in 1961 and 1962 to share news of his yoga progress and important life events and to make arrangements to meet in Europe and India. Just after his daughter Zamira's wedding to her first husband, the pianist Fou Ts'ong,[44] Menuhin had another operation at the beginning of 1961, this time for a hernia. He reported to Iyengar that he was still able to do some "exercises," and he invited Iyengar to the Bath Festival again on June 1 to give two or three demonstrations.[45] He promised to "try this time to prepare some television in advance," helpfully asked if he should arrange for transportation, and gave the family yoga report of how "Ma spent thirty minutes on her head."[46]

After knowing each other for nearly a decade, Menuhin and Iyengar developed a relationship so deeply entwined that it influenced the violinist's professional choices. As plans firmed up for Iyengar's summer trip to Europe in 1961, Menuhin knew he would be less available than the year before due to his own performance schedule. Yet he still helped to coordinate Iyengar's yoga instruction to his family and colleagues in Gstaad. Menuhin wrote: "At least Jeremy and Mme. Scaravelli [Vanda Scaravelli, a pianist and another early student of Iyengar who would go on to teach and promote yoga], and all my friends and your devoted followers will derive much pleasure and profit from your attentions."[47] Since Menuhin would not be in Gstaad until the first days of August, he suggested Iyengar first travel to London to teach, then to Brussels to be with the Queen Mother in June and July, then arrive finally in Gstaad at the end of July when Menuhin could be with him.[48]

Menuhin's support for his guru continued to strengthen Iyengar's network in Europe. Backers like Ayana Deva Angadi, founder of the Asian Music Circle, were eager for Iyengar to perform in London, and the organization established a standing arrangement with Air India to pay the round-trip fare from Bombay to Gstaad in exchange for performances under their auspices. Scaravelli, who was emerging as an important organizer for Iyengar's trips to Gstaad, had also offered to help pay the fare. Still, Menuhin wanted to protect his guru from overextension while also ensuring his high public visibility: "I feel you should not give too many performances—perhaps one television BBC performance, and one or two in London for the Circle or for Air India or perhaps one for each but I feel that your own talents should not be exploited in so poor a way as that. You must either show your ability to many thousands of people, or give your help to a chosen few."[49] Menuhin also felt concerned about equitable fees for Iyengar's work in London. When Angadi of the Asian Music Circle finally sent Iyengar one hundred pounds, Menuhin was not "too unhappy about it" but still offered to make an adjustment the next time they met in Europe.[50]

BBC INTERVIEW WITH DAVID ATTENBOROUGH: "YEHUDI MENUHIN AND HIS GURU"

While Menuhin connected Iyengar to the upper strata of European society in Switzerland, England, and Belgium, he also supported his guru's goal of reaching everyday people. As a result of those efforts, on August 21, 1963, the BBC broadcast the television program "Yehudi Menuhin and His Guru." This broadcast helped launch Iyengar into a wider audience in the West, and it captured one of the most famous moments of Menuhin and Iyengar together. Hosted by the renowned broadcaster and natural historian David Attenborough (b. 1926), the program elevated Iyengar's profile in London and boosted yoga education. In the show, Attenborough interviews Menuhin about his experiences with yoga,[51] while Iyengar joins the discussion and performs some *asanas* (see figure 3.2).

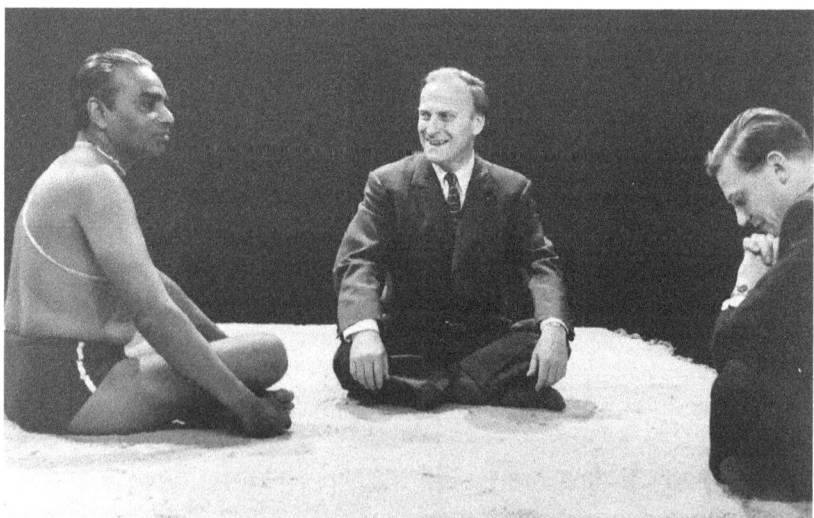

Figure 3.2. BBC program "Yehudi Menuhin and His Guru," August 21, 1963. Sitting left to right: Iyengar, Menuhin, and Attenborough. Courtesy of Foyle Menuhin Archive.

After the success of the BBC program, Iyengar began to give his first truly public classes in North London. Prashant credits Menuhin with asking Angela Marris of the Asian Music Circle to start classes under the name of the organization. Although Iyengar's first beginner's class had only five students,[52] the demand for his teaching grew so quickly that Iyengar "authorized six of his students to begin teaching in his name so they could pass on to others what he had taught them. The next year, Iyengar was back in London for six weeks to teach his new students. He returned annually thereafter."[53] As Iyengar also voyaged regularly to Switzerland to teach Menuhin in Gstaad until 1972, his teaching career continued to rise over the next twenty years through his regular trips to Europe to offer classes, demonstrations, and lectures.

LIFELONG ADVOCATE FOR IYENGAR AND YOGA

In the years that followed, Menuhin continued to demonstrate a strong commitment to his friendship with Iyengar and to advocate for yoga around the world as he aged into his sixties and seventies. In 1975, at the inauguration of RIMYI—a major milestone in Iyengar's career—Menuhin sent two messages to celebrate the occasion. He was serving as the president of the International Music Council of UNESCO at the time, and he endorsed Iyengar by writing in his official capacity: "I have known Mr. Iyengar for almost a quarter of a century and I always think of him as one of the best teachers I have ever known. I know this feeling is confirmed by all his disciples, not only among you in his home country, but all over the world."[54] Menuhin also marked the great occasion of RIMYI's inauguration in a longer personal message, where he reflected on his own yoga experiences and conveyed how the principles of the discipline integrated with his own personal philosophy. Menuhin explicitly referred to Iyengar as his "yoga guru" and credited him for spreading yoga as a means to help heal a broken world and restore balance in mind and body. His words have a haunting resonance nearly fifty years later:

> Since I first went to India at the invitation of Prime Minister Jawaharlal Nehru in 1951 [the trip was actually in 1952], a vast movement in all parts of the world has acknowledged the physical and moral properties of yoga. The ancient practice has brought a discipline of mind and body to a material and extrovert humanity, reaching the limits of its own and nature's

expendable energies. . . . We are depleting our reserves of spirit, health, courage, faith, and inner balance, at least in the ambitious countries, at an alarming rate. The quiet practice of Yoga is in its humble yet effective way an antidote.[55]

In the last two decades of his life, Menuhin also continued to endorse Iyengar's published works, even as their personal connection and correspondence became more sporadic. Menuhin wrote two additional forewords for Iyengar's books *Light on Pranayama* (1981) and *Light on the Yoga Sutras* (1993), both of which indicate his ongoing engagement with yoga and his broad view of the discipline through the work of his guru. In the foreword to *Light on Pranayama*, Menuhin highlights the virtues and benefits of practicing breath control. He says that Iyengar has placed in the layman's hands a book that contains more information, knowledge, and wisdom that represents an approach to health through an understanding of body, mind, and spirit. Menuhin's concluding statement relates his core value of "unity in diversity" to yoga: "With this book, Mr. Iyengar, my guru in yoga, has added a new and greater dimension to the life of the people of the West, urging us to join our brothers of every colour and every creed in the celebration of life with due reverence and purpose."[56] In the foreword to *Light on the Yoga Sutras*, which is Iyengar's interpretation of yoga philosophy through his translation and commentary on Patañjali's *Yoga Sutras*, Menuhin commends Iyengar as his own teacher and one of yoga's best exponents today. Menuhin broadly describes yoga as a practical art and science with a vision of human perfection of body, mind, and soul, free of any attachment to a particular religion and accessible to all people. "Anyone can practice yoga, and this important contribution to the history of yoga and its validity today is for everyone."[57]

World Music Projects and Performance

An important tenet of the Yoga of Action that Menuhin learned from Iyengar includes a selfless engagement with the world. Although Menuhin had long been involved in humanitarian work because of his natural disposition, the ethics he learned from his parents, and the traumas of World War II, his work with Iyengar and his commitment to yoga nevertheless brought a new consciousness to this kind of activity. Menuhin pursued a number of musical activities focused on cultural exchange and the alleviation of problems in the world during the early and mid-1960s. During this time of increased cultural awareness and activity, he also became a great advocate for world music, as when he invited his Indian colleagues and African musicians to perform with the Commonwealth Arts Festival in 1965. In a letter he sent to Iyengar, Menuhin expressed sympathy for Iyengar's country, presumably about political problems in India during the Indo-Pakistani War of 1965, and his concern for the state of the world: "It is all so unnecessary, as all stupid things are, but as these are in the majority, I suppose the world will never change."[58]

As a professional performer he embraced new musical traditions beyond the standard classical canon in cross-cultural encounters. In particular, his early fascination with improvisation and non-classical music during his childhood encounters with gypsy music in Romania resurfaced as he explored both Indian music and jazz. He collaborated with musicians of equal stature in these respective styles, including sitarist Ravi Shankar (1920–2012) and violinist Stéphane Grappelli (1908–1997).

INDIAN CULTURAL PROJECTS

By the mid-1960s, fifteen years since he first began his yoga practice, Menuhin became more absorbed in his new projects and plans, especially those related to Indian music and culture. He released the recording *West Meets East* with Ravi Shankar, and he also maintained his friendships with important Indian politicians, including Indira Gandhi, the prime minister at that time. After a busy summer and fall in 1966, Menuhin settled into a four-month break from recording and concerts so he could concentrate on his Indian cultural projects and writing. He was beginning to envision a television project on India, an idea that must have been forming in his mind the previous summer in Gstaad, but now he felt he must attend to other concerns, primarily helping Diana as she recovered from an illness. He described this big idea to Iyengar: "I had, as I told you, dreamed of doing some work with you at this period, but I soon realized that now I must help and maintain rather than be helped and taught. Perhaps, if I feel I have fulfilled a good part of my tasks sometime in March? But, this is still only a dream."[59] His yoga practice nevertheless continued unabated. In this same letter, Menuhin reported to Iyengar "except for momentary lapses, I have kept up the progress of last time when you were here in Gstaad and trust that I shall not disappoint you too much by the time we next meet," and he closed this letter with sentiments that reflect his continued deep caring, concern, and fondness for his guru: "I bless you every day, and pray that you and your family are well and happy in spite of the tremendously difficult and frightening times we live in. Please always tell me if I can help in some way."[60]

In 1966, John Culshaw, the head of music programming of BBC Television, approached Menuhin about doing two one-hour films on India. He asked Menuhin for a "personal evaluation, personal comment on what [he found] most striking, most valuable, most important for our world and in particular our Western world."[61] Menuhin seemed to jump at the opportunity to do this project. As he began to sketch out ideas for what he would like to show about Indian culture, philosophy, and religion, he turned to his friend Prime Minister Indira Gandhi, who he had met on his first trip to India in 1952. He told Gandhi he would also write to Ravi Shankar and his guru Iyengar about the program and asked her to help identify other people who could guide him. Although Menuhin wrote to Iyengar with the copy of the letter to Gandhi that outlined his initial ideas, I don't believe this project ever came to fruition or that Iyengar contributed to its development (at least I have found no reference to it in the BBC archive list). Still, Menuhin's idea for such a project, and the record of his initial thinking about how to approach it, reflects how deeply his yoga practice led him to become absorbed in Indian culture and "the discipline of body, mind, and breath."[62]

Menuhin may have been on a research mission for the BBC project during his fourth trip to India in 1969. Although I have found no correspondence between Menuhin and Iyengar specifically discussing this trip or more on the BBC project, Menuhin's actions—contacting both the prime minister of India and Iyengar and possibly Shankar—demonstrate how deeply he had fallen in love with the spirit and culture of India. They also reflect how strongly yogic principles had worked their way into his thinking and being, many of which he articulated in his own writings on philosophical and spiritual matters in later years.

INDIAN MUSIC AND RAVI SHANKAR

As Menuhin integrated his yoga practice and enchantment with Indian music in the 1950s and 1960s, he embodied the path of the Yoga of Action as a performer perhaps most directly through the art of improvisation. Menuhin, who always "thirsted for abandon," discovered that as "yoga promised release from physical impediments, so improvisation promised abandon to musical impulse."[63] Although he humbly called himself a "crank" in the practice of improvisation, he viewed it to be yoga in musical action.[64] Just as the practice of yoga removes obstacles to the true self, Menuhin believed that a musician must clear a channel for the Divine Spirit to flow while improvising. Yoga and improvisation were like two sides of the same coin in his quest for musical liberation.

As a performing musician, it is perhaps not surprising that Menuhin would channel his practice of the Indian discipline of yoga into the music of the country. He fell in love with Indian music when he first met his "Indian colleagues," and he was fascinated by their instruments, especially how they adapted the Western violin.[65] In particular, Menuhin actualized his yoga-centered beliefs in unity and diversity, and his value on improvisation in performance, by collaborating with the great Indian musicians Ravi Shankar, Ali Akbar Khan (1922–2009, veena and sarod), and Chatur Lal (1925–1965, tabla).

Just as Menuhin's relationship with Iyengar deepened his connection to yoga, his personal bond with Ravi Shankar strongly linked him to Indian music. Four years younger than Menuhin, Shankar had also been a child prodigy, and he had even heard Menuhin perform when they were both living in Paris in 1934.[66] When the two met as adults in India in 1952, Shankar's musicality and personality enchanted Menuhin, and the two immediately established a close connection. The brilliant Indian sitarist and composer profoundly impacted Menuhin's exploration and understanding of the "fascinating, highly evolved, and refined music of India," and Menuhin felt indebted to Shankar for "some of the most inspiring moments" of his life.[67] As with his yoga guru Iyengar, Menuhin humbly opened himself to learning from Shankar like a musical guru, and Shankar in turn reinforced Menuhin's overarching belief in the principle of unity in diversity by finding common principles in Eastern and Western music. Menuhin wrote: "Ravi Shankar has brought me a precious gift. Through him I have added a new dimension to my experience of music—one which belongs to all great music, including our own, but which, along with so much that should remain inspired and intuitive, is blueprinted out of our world."[68] Later in life, Menuhin humbly reflected on his great fortune to study and play with Shankar and how other musicians followed: "I was, of course, merely a modest successor of Ruth St. Denis and Pavlova—but by my time it was possible to be a respectful pupil of a great teacher, Ravi Shankar, and to play, however simply, authentic Indian classical music. I was followed in this by George Harrison, John Coltrane, and others. The experience remains one of the most enriching and fascinating of my life. I did not learn formulas, I lived in Ravi's imagination."[69]

On Menuhin's last trip to India in 1998, he conveyed a message to be read at a special evening tribute to Shankar in New Delhi. The violinist paid homage to his musical soulmate as he addressed how Shankar and Indian music encapsulated Indian mysticism: "You have known the whole gamut of life, from its deepest shadows to its revealing lights. You inspire us as you carry us through every human emotion, and you enable your listener to become a better human being as he or she listens, learns and shares in the perfection of your ecstasy. Through you, mystic India and the Indian pulsating heart join to draw us into another world totally different from the one we think we know."[70]

The following day, Menuhin was to appear as a guest conductor for the Lakshminarayana Global Music Festival in New Delhi, a musical tribute to the fiftieth year of Indian independence. Slated to feature ensembles from around the world, the concert signified one of Menuhin's last multicultural performance opportunities. However, as Menuhin indicated to Iyengar in a letter, his concerts for this celebration were canceled at the last minute by the Indian government.[71]

Menuhin promoted Indian music in the West as enthusiastically as he promoted yoga and Iyengar. During the 1950s and 1960s especially, Menuhin zealously introduced Shankar through various performance channels, including concerts, festivals, and TV and radio broadcasts the US and the UK. At times, Menuhin himself also participated actively as a performer of Indian music.

As early as spring 1955, Menuhin began to organize performances and programs featuring Indian music and culture, and he often delivered introductory comments. In April of that year, he first brought Shankar and Khan, along with the dancer Shanta Rao, to New York, where they performed a concert at the Museum of Modern Art and for the arts-and-culture network TV show *Omnibus*.[72] Afterward, Menuhin drafted a proposal to bring Shankar, Lal, Khan, and another tambura player on a US tour to offer performances, lectures, and demonstrations at universities, museums, and other prospective community gatherings. The proposal included all the logistics of how such a tour could work, but I don't believe it ever came to fruition.

Menuhin first introduced Indian music at the Bath Festival in 1959, and he continued that tradition for several years. The most memorable Bath Festival with Shankar was in 1966 when Menuhin performed with his Indian colleagues. Menuhin had asked Shankar to compose a piece they could play together, which he called *West Meets East*. Shankar's quid pro quo was a joint concert where Menuhin performed a Bach solo violin sonata, followed by a performance by the Indian musicians, and then for the finale "West would join East in a specifically chosen raga to suit [Menuhin's] inexperience."[73] As much as Menuhin idealized the freedom in the art of improvisation, it frightened him to actually do it. Just to be secure, he notated some of his parts in the ragas in advance of the performance with Shankar (see figures 3.3a and 3.3b).

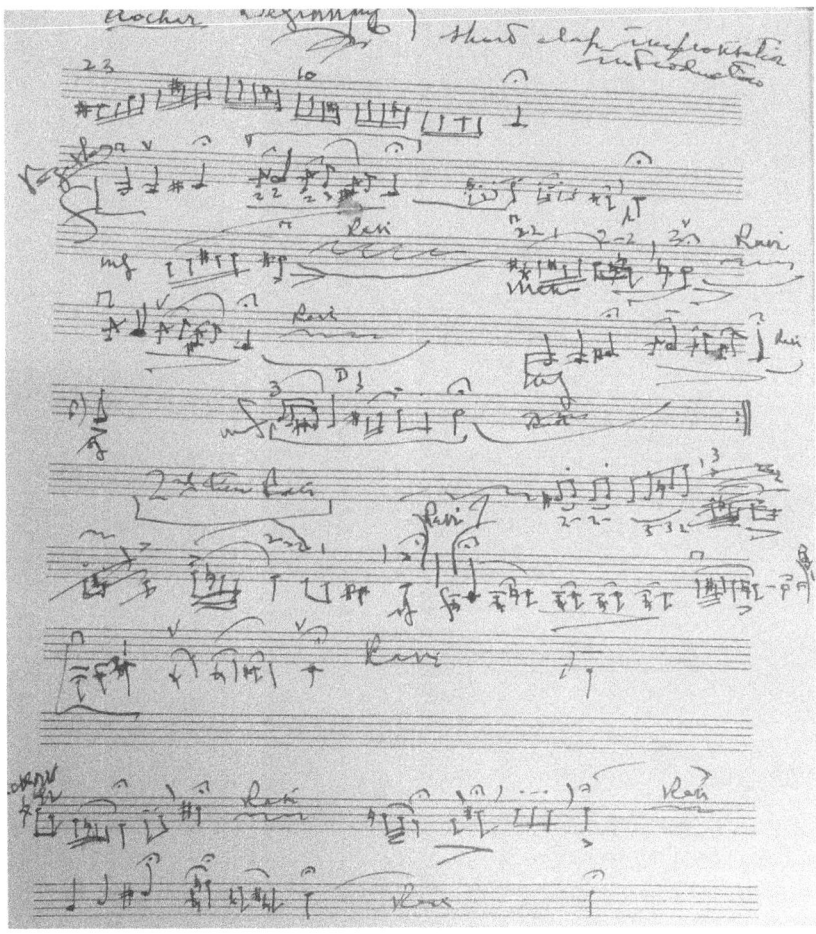

Figure 3.3a. Menuhin's music manuscript of a raga. Courtesy of Foyle Menuhin Archive.

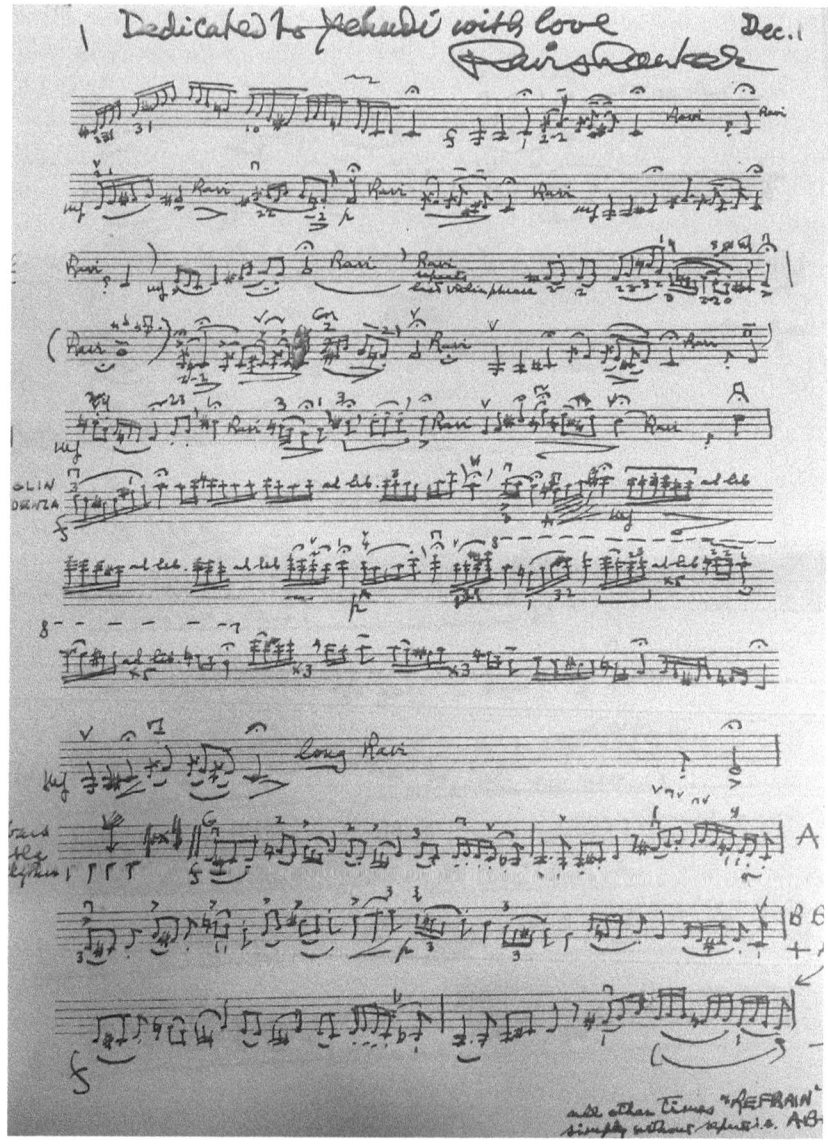

Figure 3.3b. Shankar's manuscript of a raga and inscription to Menuhin. Courtesy of Foyle Menuhin Archive.

Menuhin recalls: "Ravi Shankar's appearance at the 1966 festival briefly transformed our quarters at the Lansdowne Hotel into a corner of Old Delhi, and confronted me with one of the most scarifying challenges of my life."[74] Menuhin dressed the part as well. He walked out on stage barefoot and played in the lotus position while sitting with Shankar and Lal on the traditional Indian rugs. Upon Menuhin's entrance into the musical texture, Diana recalls: "At first Yehudi modestly played his melody and then, gathering spirit and speed from Ravi, let himself go till all three—Ravi, Chatur, and Yehudi—were tearing through a conversational trio that carried the audience away until at the end they rose and called for more."[75]

The recording *West Meets East: The Historic Shankar/Menuhin Sessions*, released soon after the memorable 1966 performance at the Bath Festival, marks one of the greatest achievements of the Menuhin-Shankar collaboration. It first appeared in Great Britain in 1966 and was then released in the US in January 1967. Bridging West and East, and in homage to his Romanian mentor, Menuhin also included Enesco's Violin Sonata No. 3 on the recording, in which his sister Hephzibah accompanied him on piano.

As Menuhin became more engaged in international service and exerted his strong humanitarian voice in the world, he brought Shankar to the UN General Assembly to perform a joint concert in 1967, which, according to Shankar, met with "thunderous success."[76] They performed *West Meets East* again "before the decade was out" at the Royal Albert Hall, where the young Prince of Wales, now King Charles III, joined them on the stage to express his admiration for Mahatma Gandhi.[77] That same year, Angadi of the Asian Music Circle, "who was also facilitating B. K. S. Iyengar's classes in Britain while in the country teaching Menuhin,"[78] introduced Shankar to George Harrison of the Beatles and arranged their first sitar lesson. Harrison, who also fell under the spell of Shankar's music, helped shuttle the sitarist into the world of popular music stardom, and in 1969 Shankar even performed at the Woodstock Music and Art Fair in New York.

Menuhin continued to promote Shankar and Indian music into the 1970s. He brought Shankar to the Windsor Festival in 1970 and to the Gstaad Festival numerous times until 1978 as well as to the Yehudi Menuhin School (discussed in detail in chapter 4) for guest classes. Just a few years before his death, Menuhin reunited with Shankar to cohost a live televised concert program from Brussels, "From the Sitar to the Guitar" in November 1995.

JAZZ AND STÉPHANE GRAPPELLI

As Menuhin continued to explore improvisation as a means to free his musical impulse in parallel with his quest to release his body from physical impediments through his yoga practice, he found another great non-classical musician with whom he could collaborate in the 1970s—the celebrated jazz violinist Stéphane Grappelli. Menuhin's interest in jazz was a natural next step for him in his search for freedom in his playing: "Ravi Shankar followed the gypsies and, in course of time, Stéphane Grappelli . . . followed Ravi Shankar, successive mentors on a journey to spontaneity."[79]

Menuhin was already acquainted with the jazz violinist's recordings when the BBC called him one Christmas morning to say he would be playing with Grappelli on his broadcast that evening, and Menuhin "finally took the plunge with the tango 'Jealousy' [sic]."[80] Menuhin connected as strongly with Grappelli as he did with Shankar. Perhaps Menuhin was able to learn and absorb even more about improvisation from Grappelli as a fellow virtuoso on the violin. Although their musical styles were different, Menuhin deeply admired the jazz violinist, "who off the cuff can use any theme to express any nuance—wistfulness, brilliance, aggression, scorn—with a speed and accuracy that stretch credulity."[81] Menuhin found the same path to musical freedom in Grappelli's jazz improvisation that he learned from his early mentor Enesco. As another example of the unity in diversity principle at work, Menuhin linked the two music styles when he wrote, "To reach our apogee, we have to subjugate our natures, then free them. In the venture, each tradition, the extempore and the interpretative, can help the other, and those musicians who synthesize the two are the most complete, the worthiest of our admiration. That is perhaps why I have always adored Enesco."[82]

Just as he brought Shankar to his school to expose students to music outside the regular classical canon, Menuhin also invited Grappelli to perform there. On one of his visits, Grappelli encountered the talented violinist Nigel Kennedy (b. 1956), who had started studying at the Menuhin School at age seven and was then in his early teens.[83] Known today as a brilliant performer who crosses between classical, jazz, and popular styles, Kennedy is one of Menuhin's most famous protégés. Kennedy had been listening carefully to Grappelli's recordings and imitating them before the elder jazz violinist's visit. When Grappelli saw Kennedy's enthusiasm for jazz, he helped mentor the teenager by taking him out to hear live jazz in clubs and even performing with him.

Menuhin's quest for freedom in his body to improve the mechanics of violin playing that initially led him to yoga also led him in other directions on the path of *karmayoga*. His pioneering work as a performer, conductor, and impresario during the 1950s, 1960s, and 1970s brought world music to Western classical audiences.[84] And Menuhin's commitment to transcending cultural boundaries with audiences and other musicians led him to explore Indian music and improvisation. Menuhin best summarizes his contributions to promoting world music with characteristic humility. For him it was "a privilege . . . to bring Indian music, art, dance and sculpture and painting to the United States for the first time," and he gratefully credited all the organizations that supported his educational mission "that enabled American people to see and hear the greatest Indian musicians, Ali Akbar Khan, Ravi Shankar, Chatur Lal, and their wonderful dancers, Shanta Rao in particular."[85]

Chapter 4

Yoga Path of Knowledge

Menuhin's Teachings and Writings

The previous chapter reflected on how yoga principles influenced Menuhin's professional activities beyond his relationship with Iyengar along the path of the Yoga of Action. Like his musical performances and organization of festivals can be understood to embrace aspects of *karmayoga*, the Yoga of Action, Menuhin's yoga-influenced studies of violin pedagogy and Indian music can be understood to embrace aspects of the path of *jñanayoga*, the Yoga of Knowledge. He transmitted the integrated music-yoga knowledge he gleaned from his yoga practice on these subjects through his teaching and writing, reflecting the dimension of the mind. Thus, during the most active years of Iyengar and Menuhin's relationship, yoga influenced not only the violinist's work as a performing musician but also his work as an educator and disseminator of knowledge.

Menuhin was an "idea man" who had the uncanny ability to communicate his educational visions to talented administrators who could help realize them. With such organizational support, Menuhin created the Yehudi Menuhin School (YMS), instructional videos and books on violin playing, and other music programs, master classes, and competitions. A prolific writer, Menuhin also published books and articles targeted for the educated lay reader—what we would call "public scholarship" today—to reach a broader community of people beyond the elite circle of classical musicians. While he wrote on a vast array of topics including Western and world music, education, politics, and the environment,[1] his writings on Indian music are particularly relevant to this discussion of Menuhin's practice of the Yoga of Knowledge, as he not only actively performed and promoted Indian music, but he also studied its structure.

Yoga's Influence on Menuhin's Violin Playing and Teaching

While Menuhin's training of his mind to understand truth and gain self-realization is especially relevant to the yogic concept of *svadhyaya* (self-study), his pursuit of musical knowledge and its application to violin playing and teaching intersects most concretely with the eight limbs of yoga. In particular, he transferred elements of yoga *asana* and *pranayama* to his teaching methods. Both limbs helped him understand the mechanics of violin playing as he incorporated the knowledge of body and breath into his pedagogy. Just like his yoga guru Iyengar developed a teaching method that first instructs the student in body alignment and mastery of *asana*, Menuhin emphasized exact and detailed instructions for the "exercises" in his pedagogy to prepare the student's body to master a solid violin technique. Yet Menuhin's method was not rigid, as he sought to capture a fine level of subtlety in the actions of the body. His holistic approach allowed for the characteristics of each individual violinist, where "the teacher . . . must know how to temper and adjust these exercises according to the physical, psychological and emotional attributes of the pupil in front of him."[2]

His teaching also reflects the inner limbs of yoga—*dharana* (concentration), *dhyani* (meditation), and *samadhi* (absorption of the consciousness in the self)—in the mental and spiritual realms. As a true yogi, Menuhin understood how harnessing the power of concentration was the first stage of absorption to rid the mind of distractions while practicing the violin. Even as a young child, he caught himself letting his mind wander during practice sessions, and he became worried enough to pull himself out of acquiring such dangerous habits. He carried this early lesson into his own teaching, noting how each student is responsible for their own concentrated practice and that concentration is a kind of meditation: "A violinist, whether eight years old or fifty-eight, leads a solitary, meditative, ruminative life, and only he is accountable for the direction of his meditations."[3] Even later, in the 1980s, Menuhin continued to transmit his yogic approach to violin teaching. For example, in his master classes at the Manhattan School of Music in February and March 1983, he delivered many instructions for the violinist that recall the yoga philosophy of union, consciousness, and total absorption regarding the "whole body . . . where the mind belongs. . . . When you play, every level of consciousness is used, and it must all work together."[4]

At the deepest level of *samadhi*, Menuhin's ongoing practice to achieve perfection in violin playing was a means to an end, like a yogi practicing *asana* to find the spiritual state of balance and equanimity. While practice is necessary to excel in anything, a yoga practitioner more pointedly seeks to master the body through "effortless effort" of *asana* to achieve *samadhi*, as expressed in Patañjali's sutra II.47: "Perfection in an *asana* is achieved when the effort to perform it becomes effortless and the infinite being within is reached."[5] Similarly, Menuhin's quest, and what drew him to yoga in the first place, was to free the body of physical struggles in his violin playing. He sought a state of equanimity when performing, where the music flowed through him without apparent effort. After Menuhin found this state of spiritual grace, he endeavored to lead students to find it also.

THE YEHUDI MENUHIN SCHOOL

Menuhin opened his school in the fall of 1963 in London, starting with just eleven string and piano students. An early inspiration came from his visit to the Soviet Union's Central School of Music on his trip to Russia in 1945, which impressed him as "shining like a lone good deed in a war-drained Moscow."[6] Observing the Russian teaching method there first planted the seed in his mind to start something similar in the West. But not until he acquired his first protégé in the mid-1950s, the teenage Argentine violinist Alberto Lysy (1935–2009), did Menuhin's ideas for his own school begin to take root. Over a two-year period, Menuhin laid the groundwork by forming an advisory committee and fundraising. After one year in London, the school moved to a beautiful estate with two buildings in Stoke d'Abernon, Surrey, in 1964. That same year, the BBC show *Master Classes* featured students from the school, most notably Menuhin himself coaching then seven-year-old violinist Nigel Kennedy.[7]

In the formative stages of his school, Menuhin worked closely with two musical pillars: Alberto Lysy, who was then a young adult, and Marcel Gazelle, his longtime collaborative pianist. Although Lysy's budding career prevented him from teaching regularly at the school, Gazelle became its first musical director. They had designed the school to function administratively without Menuhin's hands-on presence, although he regularly taught there.

Through the years, Menuhin's broad educational mission brought in many distinguished musicians, including such renowned musicians as Itzhak Perlman and Nadia Boulanger, and other great thinkers like the economist Fritz Schumacher, author of the 1973 classic *Small Is Beautiful.*[8] By 1972, the YMS had thirty-eight students and the campus added a new third building. That same year, a neighbor restored and donated an old barn as the school's concert hall.[9] The school has continued to expand and update its facilities, including the Menuhin Hall, a three-hundred-seat concert hall built in 2006. Today, the school accommodates approximately eighty students between ages eight and nineteen, including many international students. Offering instrumental lessons in strings, guitar, piano, and voice, the faculty include regular and distinguished guest teachers. As of this writing, the renowned pianist/conductor Daniel Barenboim currently serves as president emeritus. Menuhin considered the YMS to be the crowning achievement of his life,[10] and it remains a vital educational institution for young musicians today (see figure 4.1).

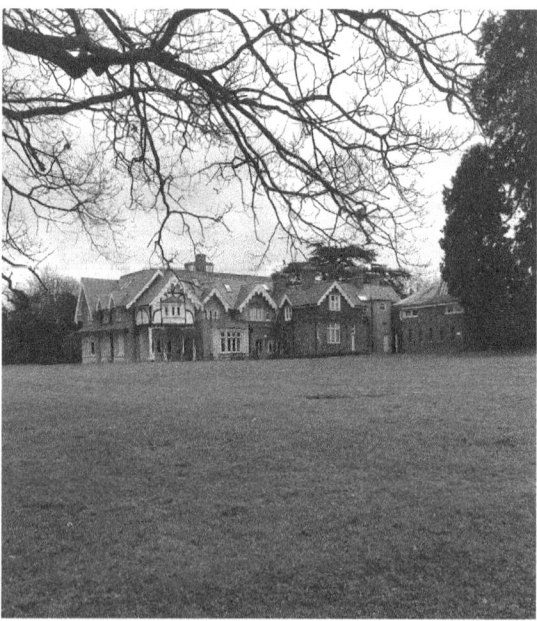

Figure 4.1. Yehudi Menuhin School. Photo by Kristin Wendland.

A true idealist in search of a kind of physical and spiritual liberation like *samadhi*, Menuhin admitted that his "life has been spent in creating Utopia."[11] Shaped by his own early musical life and training, Menuhin founded his school on principles he learned and experienced growing up—his search for utopia, the conviction that he had something unique to contribute, and a zeal to pass it on. And, like a yogi following the path of the Yoga of Knowledge, he channeled his musical knowledge and experience in a systematic way, while he integrated key elements of yoga into his educational mission. Motivated by his sense of obligation to share his knowledge, Menuhin's mission was to create a "happy, healthy community of the young."[12] He knew he had something unique to contribute from his own experience, including his lessons from yoga and even his early "collaborative laboratory" of making music with his sister Hephzibah.[13] Having "made his pilgrimage" as an adult to "comprehension of the violin," which as the Menuhin-Iyengar correspondence shows was largely guided by his yoga practice, he wanted to help others and pass on "his findings."[14]

Menuhin took a yoga-like holistic approach to his educational mission. He never intended his school to be a conservatory, but rather he sought to educate musically well-rounded young students. Taking a more flexible approach than the Russian model of training soloists, he prioritized giving students a wider array of musical training. In keeping with his values on cultivating cultural diversity, he exposed students to music beyond the Western canon early on, demonstrated by the visits from Grappelli and Shankar in the 1960s. He and his faculty "wanted to train musical all-rounders, fitted to moving on into teaching, chamber groups, orchestra, or solo work."[15] They created an atmosphere that was less competitive and more community-oriented. Menuhin believed England itself offered the perfect environment for his vision since it "is a land where the team is uppermost."[16] Still he hoped the "Gallic-Viennese-Romanian spirit" of his childhood mentor Georges Enesco presided there too, not only through himself but also through Gazelle's wife Jacqueline, who had also studied with Enesco as a child and who taught violin at the school.[17] Menuhin also broadened student performance opportunities outside of his school, both at festivals in England and on trips abroad. In addition to regular performances at the Gstaad Festival in Switzerland, YMS students traveled to other European countries, the US, China, and Israel.[18]

Menuhin based his pedagogical approach on his own study of the violin and the knowledge he acquired through years of experience, much of it directly influenced by his yoga practice with Iyengar. He never constricted it to anything he would call "the Menuhin method," yet he intentionally taught on two levels. While they reflect concepts of technique and musicality all good music teachers seek to convey, these two levels may also be understood to mirror Menuhin's yogic approach to teaching. First, he taught on the "violinistic" level to enable a student to play adequately, just as *asana* strengthens the body to function fluidly. Second, he taught on the musical level to reach the student's deeper creative spirit, just as the yogi moves beyond *asana* to reach deeper spiritual levels in meditation. In short, Menuhin pushed students beyond technical playing to use their interpretative powers and intelligence in making music—two indispensable skills for an aspiring yoga practitioner as well.

As Menuhin's core focus was always on cultivating a flexible and relaxed body, a yoga analogy again clearly aligns with his approach. Just as calming the body is the first step toward removing obstacles in the path of quieting the consciousness to realize the true self in yoga, so Menuhin sought to prepare students to realize their own vision of the music with "a sense of fluency, economy, and precision in motion."[19] He knew the student must first remove the physical obstacles blocking the ability to play freely, just as a yogi must remove obstacles blocking the true self. In order to unlock a flow of creativity, he invented exercises to develop physical coordination between the hands and also between playing the instrument and the breath to allow the student's imagination and intuition to take over.[20]

Menuhin's educational philosophy reflected yogic principles, and he naturally included actual yoga classes in the students' holistic course of study from the school's inception. One student of the first YMS graduating class provided this description about Menuhin: "Well, he has worked out this system of exercises which he originally applied to himself. And he's given them to us. It's based on relaxation, and the tension that is built up."[21] Such "exercises" were built into the daily schedule, as Menuhin describes the holistic routine:

> The children get up at 7:30, go through simple exercises based on Yoga, breakfast, and then take a run in the garden before lessons begin. These are divided into two parts. One is scholastic, and the other is musical. One-half of the children start with music first, and then continue with their academic studies and vice versa. Lunch follows according to my dietary principals of organically produced foods. It is cooked by none other than Mrs. Joachim, a descendant of the great violinist himself.[22]

Menuhin also incorporated an ecumenical practice at his school for students to tap into a spiritual energy that permeates all living things. It included communal singing to cleanse the lungs and to "join us to each other and to the cosmos," followed by an inspirational reading, and finally a period of silence to find a "stillness within."[23]

When my undergraduate research assistant at Emory University, violinist Catherine MacGregor, and I visited the school in March 2018, we had the good fortune to talk with Natasha Boyarsky, a distinguished violin teacher on the faculty. Menuhin had first met Boyarsky in Moscow, and he personally invited the Russian pedagogue to teach at his school in 1991. He trusted she would promote his approach since she "has a motherly way with very young pupils which ensures that no joints in the child's anatomy are allowed to be anything other than supple, soft, and eager to cooperate."[24] Boyarsky, who had already experienced yoga before, explained the discipline's importance in training young violin students and endorsed other benefits of yoga for musicians: "It helps to develop and keep attention, to develop control, and to feel part of your body here [in the mind]."[25]

After his death in 1999, Menuhin was buried on the school grounds. His beloved wife Diana, who died in 2003, is buried next to his grave. Menuhin's yoga practice and spiritual legacy continue to be visible on the campus today. As a tribute to Menuhin, the school installed a meditation path in 2016, the centenary of his birth, as a "calm and contemplative space that invites reflection on the spiritual and humanitarian values of Yehudi Menuhin."[26] Located in the center of the campus, the meditation path represents the importance of spiritual well-being at the school and honors Menuhin's legacy.

Menuhin's Other Educational Projects

Beyond his school, Menuhin's musical study and pursuit of knowledge yielded other fruits that exemplify how his life embodied the Yoga of Knowledge. In keeping with his guru's charge for a yogi to be of selfless service, and his commitment to the dissemination of knowledge, Menuhin founded two important projects that still flourish today. One is the European String Teachers Association, founded in 1972 at a time when Menuhin was also deeply involved in Indian music, and the other is the biannual Yehudi Menuhin International Competition for Young Violinists, established in 1983. Shortly before he died, Menuhin reiterated his holistic educational mission when he wrote of his competition's excellent record to discover and support young talent, and its aim to foster a supportive environment "to encourage cultural exchange and the development of new friendships . . . [and to] give participants the opportunity to meet and learn from one another."[27]

Menuhin's life on the path of the Yoga of Knowledge continued to reflect his values on unity, holistic training, and cultural diversity throughout the 1970s and 1980s. His most notable project, the Gstaad Academy, expanded his important work to push performers to transcend musical boundaries and cultural stereotypes. Founded in 1977 as an educational venture for young string players in transition to becoming full professionals, the Gstaad Academy followed similar educational principles as YMS by focusing on chamber, orchestral, and contemporary music. In collaboration with Alberto Lysy, his former student and now colleague, Menuhin selected sixteen international string players between the ages of seventeen and twenty-six to form a camerata or small chamber orchestra.[28] The group became a year-round extension of the summer Gstaad Festival. Following Menuhin's vision of cultural unity and using music as a means to achieve world peace, the Camerata traveled internationally to hold short residencies in European countries including Germany, Italy, and Spain and also farther abroad in Argentina, China, Japan, and the US. Still thriving today, the Gstaad Academy continues to offer a complete range of master courses addressed to young professionals, youth orchestra players, and amateur musicians of all ages.

Perhaps in recognition of his remarkable international efforts, Menuhin was named the first ever Western honorary professor of the Beijing Conservatoire in 1979, just seven years after Richard Nixon's historic trip to China that reestablished communication with the West. After the twenty-five-year break of political and diplomatic discourse, Menuhin's extraordinary honor opened the door for a cultural exchange between China and the West. Chinese students were permitted to leave their country to study at the YMS and the Menuhin Gstaad Academy, and the Camerata traveled to China in 1982.

Two violinists from the Atlanta Symphony Orchestra (ASO) worked directly with Menuhin through the Gstaad Academy in the 1980s. One of them, Lisa Yancich, went on the China tour with the group in 1982. Yancich recalled how Menuhin's commitment to disseminating knowledge exposed the young Western musicians to world music and instruments. A group boat ride on the beautiful Yangtze River was a highlight of the trip for her, where they listened to the "phenomenal" Chinese music students play their traditional instruments (see figure 4.2).[29]

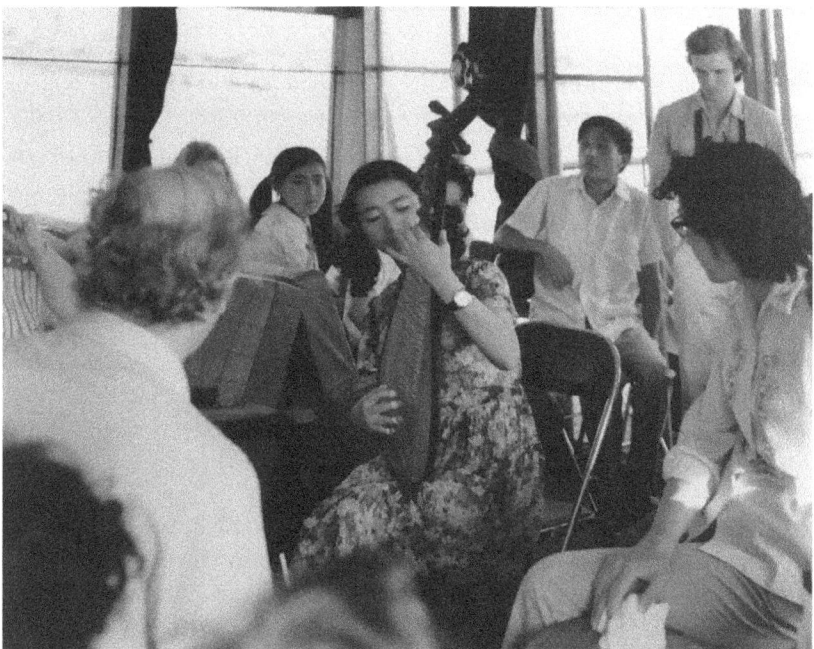

Figure 4.2. Gstaad Academy China tour, 1982. Student playing the pipa, with Menuhin facing her. Photo by Lisa Wiedman Yancich.

Another ASO violinist, Christopher Pulgram, attended the academy from 1985 to 1987, when he also recorded and toured with Menuhin. Pulgram's memories of those two years show how deeply Menuhin had assimilated his yoga practice into his life and work. The younger violinist recounted seeing Menuhin practice yoga, how the maestro recommended it to all of the students, and how he discussed its concepts and application. Pulgram also recalled how Menuhin taught academy residents not only how to play music but also how to be thoughtful and compassionate musicians:

> What was amazing about Menuhin was that the music was so personal to him. He really wanted us all to know what being an artist was; what a privilege it was and what our responsibilities were; that we were all ambassadors when we would be going from one country to the next; that we would not be playing just notes but expressing this thing that we all shared as human beings. He thought it was our duty to work toward greater understanding and compassion.[30]

MENUHIN'S BOOKS AND VIDEOS ON VIOLIN PLAYING

As Menuhin integrated yoga into his study and practice of violin playing and teaching, he captured his approach in two important books, *Violin: Six Lessons with Yehudi Menuhin* (1971) and *Life Class: Thoughts, Exercises, Reflections of an Itinerant Violinist* (1986; also published in the US under the title *The Compleat Violinist*). They present perhaps the most convincing pedagogical evidence of how yoga impacted Menuhin's approach to violin playing and also the cause-and-effect of how yoga influenced his musical life more broadly. Discussed in detail below, both books explicitly display the strong influence of Menuhin's yoga practice in all three realms of body, mind, and spirit.

VIOLIN: SIX LESSONS WITH YEHUDI MENUHIN (1971)

Menuhin first formally transmitted his yoga knowledge to violin playing in a six-part series of short films called *Violin*. Each video, filmed at the YMS, runs about twenty-five minutes, and the series includes students representing various stages of technical development. Soon after making these videos, Menuhin captured his ideas in the book *Violin: Six Lessons with Yehudi Menuhin* (see figure 4.3).

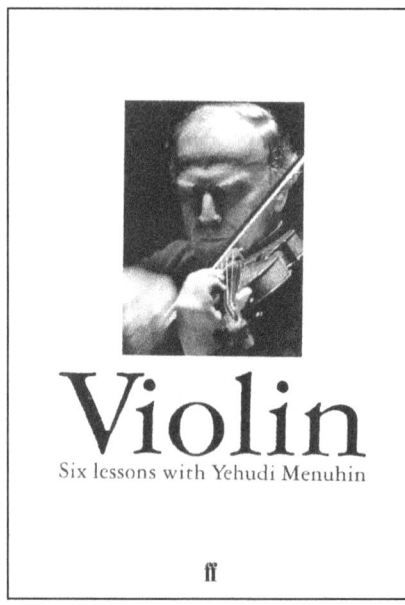

Figure 4.3. *Violin: Six Lessons* cover. Courtesy of Faber Music.

Each chapter of the book amplifies and explains the six lessons on film. In the acknowledgments, Menuhin references the impact of his yoga practice in the lessons to follow. He expresses gratitude "to the man who I sometimes call 'my best violin teacher,' Mr. B. K. S. Iyengar, my yoga guru" and that "some of the principles I have evolved are based on yoga and on his teaching of yoga and several of the exercises in the first lesson are his inspiration."[31]

As Menuhin sets the stage in the introduction for the chapters to come, he invokes many yogic principles to help master the violin. Like the same great task of a yogi to remove obstacles on the way to liberation, he points to ways to reduce "impediments of any kind" to playing the instrument, and in keeping with the principles of *niyama* and *asana*, to "cultivate an attitude of mind and heart" and "certain habits of hygiene and general physical condition."[32] He stresses the importance of the "moral attitude" (*yama*) as a "kind of bridge between the past and the future and between oneself and the outside world,"[33] where dedicated practice (*abhyasa*) in solitude leads to reward when one gives of themselves to audiences in performance (*asmita*). In addition to emphasizing how mental and physical health are crucial for a violinist to maintaining resistance and strength, Menuhin recommends a balanced diet with wholesome foods and free of sugar, cigarettes, and alcohol. In the larger view, Menuhin aims to "provide the firm underpinnings of theory, method and application" while specifying subtle details of instruction "to those minute movements, those inner feelings of parts of the fingers, which become, as it were, antennae."[34]

Before he even brings the instrument into play, Menuhin lays his foundation in "Lesson One: General Preparatory Exercises" by implicitly and explicitly referencing yoga. Menuhin's approach is based on what he calls "wave or pulse action, which reconciles conflicting impulses and directions in any one continuous activity."[35] He first wants to ensure the student has an awareness of the physical forces required for violin playing, and he describes movement in terms of ellipses, circles, and arcs. Conserving energy as momentum is essential in his approach. Menuhin captures the importance of balancing opposing forces in the body to create a point of equilibrium. He often returns to the basic idea of reconciling opposing forces, which echoes Patañjali's sutra II.48. This sutra describes how the yoga practitioner will calmly accept dualities after practicing asana with "effortless effort." Menuhin writes: "The wave action not only reconciles opposing forces by its ebb and flow, but also holds within itself the alternation of the active impulse and the passive momentum, the alternation of tension and relaxation. Within each cycle of movement there is moment of minimum effort and a point of perfect balance—I would call it the zero point."

Menuhin explicitly integrates concepts and techniques from the yoga limbs *asana* and *pranayama* in his preparatory exercises, although he never refers directly to the Sanskrit names. As in yoga, where a practitioner must first gain strength and control of the body before venturing into the realms of concentration, meditation, and total absorption, Menuhin introduces the violin student to techniques for training the body and controlling the breath as a foundation for mastering the violin. Menuhin understood how the breath (*prana*) is the energizing life force, and he stresses how "it is essential to be aware of it while practicing."[36] He defines good breathing as the ability to inhale and exhale evenly over as long a period as possible, and he offers breath exercises right out of traditional *pranayama* instructions. For example, his illustrative diagram 1 shows digital breathing, where the practitioner alternately inhales and exhales through the right and left nostrils in a thin column of air while gently closing the other nostril.[37]

Menuhin carefully explains the supreme importance of good posture as an essential foundation of violin playing exactly like a yoga teacher would explain how to practice *asana*. While it may appear that a yoga practitioner is passively holding a static pose, a good teacher provides instructions for the tremendous amount of internal work required to balance actions in some parts of the body with relaxation in others. Likewise, Menuhin stresses how one must discover a natural stance that will "absorb and accommodate the various movements of the body associated with playing the violin."[38] Just holding the violin can present the student with obstacles. The student must be able to hold the instrument in a natural posture to allow true freedom of movement and the ability to continuously adjust movements, which he emphasizes is the "secret of violin playing."[39]

Like a good yogi, Menuhin directs the student to perform these exercises barefoot. He first directs the student to find the correct center of weight on the balls of the feet, and he essentially reframes Iyengar's instructions for the foundational *tadasana* (Mountain Pose) as the basis for good posture. His diagram 2 also illustrates the internal energy flow a student should try to feel throughout the body from the foundation in the feet to the head. Next, Menuhin outlines a series of stretching and balancing exercises, including what he calls "the stork" done on one leg. His "swinging exercises" prepare movements for playing the violin. They call on his emphasis of continuous motion to stretch the arms, torso, shoulders, and back. To conclude his preparatory chapter, Menuhin identifies five basic yoga postures with instructions and diagrams, the first four to be coordinated with three cycles of the breath: Prayer Pose behind the back (*paschima namaskarasana*), Shoulder Stand Pose (*sarvangasana*), Plough Pose (*halasana*), Bridge Pose (*setubandha sarvangasana*), and Corpse Pose (*savasana*). Notably, Shoulder Stand Pose and Corpse Pose are two sequential postures that typically conclude an Iyengar Yoga class.

To Menuhin, "violin playing is an art of self-discovery,"[40] and in the following five chapters he lays out his approach to actually playing the violin. Still, his instructions echo and build on his yoga-based exercises in the preparatory chapter as he addresses techniques for holding the bow in the right hand, holding the violin in the left hand and shoulder, practicing bow movements and left-hand movements, and playing with both hands together. Throughout his lessons Menuhin emphasizes ways to release tension, and he shows how to maintain flexibility, balance, coordination, and integration in the body. He summarizes his holistic approach to violin playing in lesson 6 in a reverential tone: "Like love which requires two to become one, so violin playing only becomes alive with the complete integration and co-ordination of both hands. To achieve this state (in which the breathing also plays an essential part), the whole of the upper body must itself be flexibly, yet firmly poised, ready to yield to and to reconcile, as well as to initiate and maintain the movements."[41]

Finally, in appendix I, Menuhin offers six hints on practicing, where he again calls on his yoga experience of physical practice and self-study (*svadhyaya*). Specifically, he advises the student to never clench the jaw (a standard yoga instruction, too!), concentrate on the breath, pause and return to a state of relaxation after exerting effort, and focus the mind on concurrent details so to be "continually active, checking detail after detail."[42]

Life Class (The Compleat Violinist): Thoughts, Exercises, Reflections of an Itinerant Violinist

Fifteen years after publishing *Violin: Six Lessons*, Menuhin worked out many of his yoga-related ideas in his approach to violin playing in *Life Class*. His second book moves beyond a narrow focus on violin training as it weaves together a narrative about Menuhin's life as a musician, his "exercises" for the body, his violin technique, and many of his ideas about music. Throughout the four chapters—"An Introduction," "On Tour," "On Composers and Performers," and "Fiddler on the Hoof"—Menuhin intersperses vignettes on musical topics with a series of six exercises accompanied by photos of his own demonstrations. In these exercises, Menuhin continually returns to the theme of integration of body and motion in small and subtle actions for playing the violin, and he emphasizes aware-ness of the bodily space a violinist embraces when playing the instrument.

Throughout the work, Menuhin intertwines his knowledge and expe-rience gleaned from yoga in subtle and direct ways. He especially echoes concepts from key yoga *sutras* regarding "effortless practice" as he presents ways to help a violinist free the body of physical limitations that block the creative flow. Just as yoga can remove obstacles in a practitioner's con-sciousness in order to "abide in one's true nature," Menuhin's exercises are intended to help violinists remove obstacles to their violin technique in order to achieve true musical expression of the self. While Menuhin emphasizes concepts and techniques from *asana* and *pranayama* like in his first book, he also touches on principles and concepts essential to the other six limbs of yoga—*yama, niyama, pratyahara, dharana, dhyana,* and *samadhi*—although again never by their Sanskrit names. In this more personal and reflective work, Menuhin reveals deeper levels of integration of yoga and music as he touches on many themes related to his philosophical/spiritual belief system (which are discussed in detail in chapter 5).[43]

Beginning with characteristic honesty and humility in the first chapter, Menuhin lets the reader know his work is not intended to be a strict method, but rather he intends to share the knowledge gained from his quest to understand the body in relation to his instrument. He only wishes "to set down experiences and exercises as they have crucially affected the only violinist I feel I can comment on with any authority—myself."[44] Yogic concepts and philosophy jump off the page as Menuhin describes his approach to violin playing—words and phrases such as "equilibrium" (*sattva*); the "body moving in harmony" (union); "continuous refinement" (*abhyasa*); "search for enlightenment and harmony" (*samadhi*); and how the mind must "continuously engage in routine checking to improve aware-ness" (*svadhyaya*). Similar to acquiring a *siddhi* (yogic power), Menuhin promises that upon discovering they are on the right path of heightened awareness and sensitivity, violinists will find "greater joy, greater elation, greater abandonment, [and] greater freedom. . . . The effects will be felt in the musician and . . . also in the music, for the music will become a carrier of the musician's own inner harmony. As he or she improves, so the music's compelling, convincing, persuasive powers will increase in the same proportion."[45] As in *Violin: Six Lessons*, Menuhin includes yoga-based preparatory activities at the end of the introduction in exercise 1, including special attention to the feet and toes, stretching, and breathing.

In chapter 2, "On Tour," Menuhin refers to yoga concepts as he reflects on his busy life as a traveling musician for over fifty years. He relished the solitude of being "incarcerated" in hotel rooms, where he could be free of the "tyranny of time" and able to deeply concentrate (*dharana*) and find total absorption (*samadhi*) in preparing for concerts.[46] Ever mindful of what he put into his body, Menuhin again stressed the importance of maintaining a clean diet free of sugar, alcohol, white bread, and desserts. "A Violinist's Shopping List" includes foods and other items like herbal teas and bath essences he considered vital while on tour.[47]

In this chapter Menuhin also includes demonstrations of actual yoga poses as well as his own adaptions of yoga-like movements targeted for the violinist to achieve fluid body motions. Following his warm-up techniques of bending and stretching, relaxing the neck, and balancing on the feet in exercise 2, he instructs and illustrates how to execute such standard yoga *asanas* as Downward Facing Dog Pose (what he calls "the press up"), Shoulder Stand Pose, Plough Pose, and Head Stand Pose. Then in exercise 3, Menuhin explains his own techniques that he calls "painting" and "golf swing" to promote freedom of movement in the arms, and he offers instructions in other standard yoga postures well-suited to violinists, such as "working behind the back" (*gomukasana*) and what he now calls "fiddler's prayer" (*paschima namaskarasana*, see figure 4.4). Finally, Menuhin applies his exercises to the violin with "shadow fiddling," specifically related to holding an imaginary violin and the bow.

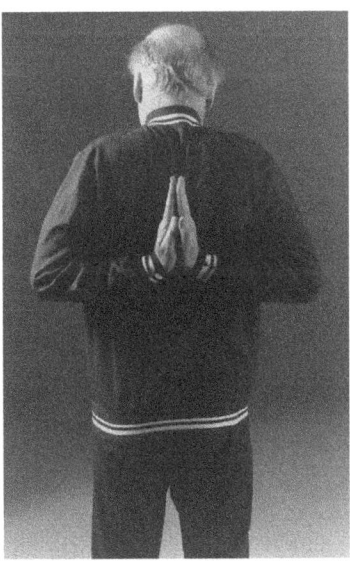

Figure 4.4. Menuhin in "fiddler's prayer." Photo by Malcolm Crowther. Courtesy of ArenaPAL.

Menuhin's deeper yoga values surface in chapter 3, "On Composers and Performers." Even as he reflects on performing and interpreting the music of various composers from Bach and Beethoven to Bartók and Enesco, he muses on more philosophical issues. For example, in his reflections "On the Violinist," Menuhin suggests universal yogic values like *ahimsa* (non-harming) as he discusses how artistry finds balance and subtlety in a world full of violence and barbarity, and how "true art teaches instead humility, tolerance, honour, and respect."[48] As the ASO violinist Christopher Pulgram observed in the maestro's teaching at the Gstaad Academy, Menuhin's own words express his belief in the duty of the musician to spread compassion through music. Even more, they express his fundamental belief in how such "enlightened human behavior" also applies to violin playing, and therefore he "looks upon music as the most complete exposition of the body and spirit of man—of our universe."[49]

Menuhin's yoga-centered approach pervades the preliminary exercises in this chapter as he teaches interdependence of all parts of the body and how "no movement happens in isolation."[50] As he discusses the bow in exercise 4, Menuhin asks the violinist to use her powers of observation (*svadhyaya*) while doing the actions of an upbow and downbow. Like a true yogi, he infuses a spiritual quality to these instructions through the word "surrender," which helps the practitioner let go of tension, while also linking the motion to the breath (*pranayama*). Menuhin's instructions are demonstrated for "taking up the bow," "strengthening exercises," and "the push and the pull."

Menuhin's cleverly titled final chapter, "Fiddler on the Hoof," conveys many other ways he integrated yoga into his life and teaching. In the opening narrative about his life as a traveling musician, he promotes a yogic-centered approach as he incorporates principles of the *niyamas*. For example, in dealing with critics Menuhin maintains *santosa* (contentment) as he humbly encourages "an attitude of acceptance and even gratitude" for both positive and negative lessons that reviews may teach a performer.[51] In one short paragraph titled "Against Drink and Drugs," he upholds his values of the *niyama sauca* (cleanliness) as a means to prevent one of the nine yoga disturbances, *bhranti darsana* (living under an illusion). He advocates keeping the body clean as he warns the performer against "anything that provides an illusion of assurance. Such false comforters have proved the undoing of many a great artist."[52]

Menuhin's discourse on "nerves and stage fright" echoes the yogic practice of identifying and dealing with obstacles (yoga *klesas*) as he shares his experience of handling this bane of the performing musician. In a kind of karmic cause-and-effect framework, he stresses how it is "important to know that such an affliction is an end product, not a first cause."[53] Menuhin categorizes three such afflictions, namely technical problems, emotional tension, and fear, and he offers remedies for each.

First, violinists must face the physical obstacles in the body that cause problems in their technique. Menuhin's remedy to have "faith in work over a very prolonged period"[54] strongly echoes Patañjali's sutra I.14, "Long, uninterrupted, alert practice is the firm foundation for restraining the fluctuations."[55] Furthermore, Menuhin's insistence that a great deal of effort is required to master technique "to render it effortless"[56] reframes sutra II.47: "Perfection in an asana is achieved when the effort to perform it becomes effortless and the infinite being within is reached."[57] Then, like the promise in yoga to find liberation, Menuhin describes the rewards of recognizing and correcting technical deficiencies. A continuous stream of integrated attention (*dhyana*) will result "when musician and music are joined in one even flow of body, mind, will, and imagination in which everything is correct and continuous."[58] Menuhin's promise again echoes a yoga sutra, III.2, which states how "a steady, continuous flow of attention directed towards the same point or region is meditation (*dyyana*)."[59]

The second affliction, emotional tension during performance, presents more difficult hindrances in violin playing. Menuhin's solution to calming such worries is to shore up concentration (*dharana*) in the mind and stay in the present moment. Then the performer may be free "to do his job . . . to translate what he sees in a composition, the ideal image of the score, into sound."[60] In short, the end result is a kind of *samadhi*, where the emotions of the performer flow unencumbered into the music.

Fear, arguably a complex and fraught issue for performers, presents a third psychological obstacle to many musicians, especially fear of failure and inadequacy. Although this is not always easy to accomplish, Menuhin encourages a performer to detach (*vairagya*) from such fears by removing the ego and letting go of outcomes in a performance. "The performer must give everything to the work; but he must not be dominated by it, he must not allow himself to be subject to one single exclusive dominant ambition or fear."[61] Menuhin suggests the way to counter the fear of memory lapses is to practice mental discipline, again concentration, by going through the musical scores in one's head.[62]

Menuhin concludes this exposition on facing nerves and stage fright by stressing the importance of rest and relaxation to calm the spirit. For him, yoga was a key to maintaining such inner peace. He acknowledges how, although he played the violin well when he was young, he did not really know how to play it. He remembers often being in a state of exhaustion or excitement, but as he later "became interested in yoga and other exercises as a means of developing a feeling of inner calm," he learned how aging solo performers must "pace themselves and conserve energy—or they will crack beneath the strain."[63]

Menuhin lays out his yoga-centered approach for handling the violin in the final two sets of exercises in chapter 4 as he continually reinforces how to maintain an awareness of movement and its cause-and-effect. Three examples in exercise 5 demonstrate his approach, namely "putting up the violin," "the pivot of the elbow," and "rolling the violin." Menuhin then calls upon a couple of key yogic concepts in the section "Some Warming Up Exercises." As if beginning an *asana* class, he starts gently and progresses to more intensity by degrees as he encourages the violinist to develop heightened awareness of the fingers. To aid in focusing the mind, Menuhin instructs how to coordinate the breath while humming on an exhalation. This is an actual *pranayama* technique called *bhramari* breath (like a buzzing bee).

Two yogic-centered bowing exercises follow in exercise 5. "Bowing but not scraping" subtly breaks down the order of component parts of bowing into active motions and relaxation. "Rhythmic pressures on the bow" recommends continued observation of body movements, always with an eye to integrate them. His relevant paragraph on wrist flexibility further instructs about the cause-and-effect of an integrated arm and wrist action, where a firm, though not rigid, "wrist and the base of the thumb (which is a crucial pivot) remains receptive to the momentum from the arm."[64]

Menuhin intersperses his practical exercises with other yoga-centered words of encouragement to the aspiring violinist. In his final exercise 6, he first reminds the violinist to approach practice holistically, as "one is dealing with a living entity," and to remember that "every action has its reaction."[65] As he deliberately touches on spiritual matters, Menuhin encourages the violinist to have faith in oneself and in the process of motion:[66] "You must have faith in the motion and faith in the continuity of the motion—faith that it will carry you provided you go with it and not against it, and provided that through practice the trajectories along which the motion flows are perfected."[67]

Back to more practical matters, Menuhin points the violinist to finger dexterity in "aiming for flexibility of thumb and fingers exercises," followed by his "finger exercises." Menuhin relays his yogic body/mind perspective of how the player must relax and let go of tension in order to accomplish these actions. Invoking yet another core yoga concept of non-attachment (*vairagya*), he acknowledges how the natural human tendency is to "hold, to grasp, to cling to things. But this involves tension—and tension shortens the muscles. The result is loss of flexibility, a holding back, a fear—which has a bad effect on the playing."[68] To conclude these finger exercises, Menuhin again sounds like a yoga instructor encouraging the violinist to release, let go, and practice: "The violinist should be the least grasping of creatures. He or she has to learn to give, to open, to lift. These lifting and falling exercises, assiduously practiced, will give a very resilient, spring-like action to the fingers."[69] Menuhin then demonstrates a good way to check one's hand position in "shifting."

Writing as a musician who ultimately absorbs himself in the sense of sound, Menuhin concludes his instructions by offering suggestions for the violinist to control and study vibrato in his "note on vibrato." Menuhin frames his approach to this basic violin technique in keeping with the yogic self-study practice of *svadhyaya* as articulated by Iyengar and other modern yoga gurus: "The violinist must learn to control every possible nuance of tone. It is a question of sensitivity, of subtlety, of learning to know yourself." On the pure level of sound, he summarizes the benefits of his exercises and how they "point towards the possibility of sensing and welcoming these vibrations."[70] Finally, he reminds the student/reader that when practicing the violin, she should always move from soft to loud, and from slow to fast, by degrees. Again like practicing *asana*, this instruction prompts the student to begin a practice session gently and then gradually demand more from the body.

Menuhin encapsulates many aspects of yoga philosophy as he brings a spiritual perspective to his views on life and music in the conclusion of *Life Class*, "Images of the Self: Some Final Thoughts." A violinist must draw on the imagination (*vikalpa*) to build a positive self-image and to visualize results of motions and actions. Again, this requires pure concentration with an eye on non-harming (*ahimsa*), rather than forcing oneself with a strong will into practicing hours, for "brutality has no place in the life of the violin."[71] Menuhin inspires hope by describing the fruits of such practice: "By analysis and cool development of subtle sensations I find that I have improved the quality of my sound, reduced tension, acquired greater precision and expression of pitch, liberated my musical inspiration and worked less."[72] His goal is to clear a channel for creative energy to flow by bringing the whole body into practice, to acquire the "readiness to express oneself, and that can happen only when all the avenues are clear."[73] Finally, as a true yogi, Menuhin invokes equanimity, detachment, and self-study in both life and work: "I advocate that in the handling of any problem in life one should aim for a balance, remaining sensitively responsive, analytical and pragmatic, with an attitude both critical and encouraging."[74] *Life Class* represents Menuhin's lifelong search for these qualities, and he dedicates it to "all his colleagues, young and old, in the hope that I may spare them time and trouble (though not effort and thought) and that they may thus be allowed to give and receive joy and wisdom, support and help in more abundant measure."[75]

Menuhin's Knowledge and Advocacy of Indian Music

While yoga led Menuhin to actively engage with Indian music as a performer on the path of the Yoga of Action, his curious mind led him to study its musical structure and how it might connect to Western music on the path of the Yoga of Knowledge. And just as he shared his yoga-influenced approach to teaching and violin playing, he sought to disseminate his knowledge of Indian music to the general reader and audience. An underlying current of idealism consistently runs throughout his writings on the subject, along with his strong moral convictions about life and his spiritual belief in "unity in diversity." These spiritual convictions radiate Menuhin's burning zeal to advocate for and share knowledge of Indian music in particular.

Menuhin felt he had much to learn from the ancient culture of India, especially Indian music, after he started to practice yoga. He first went to India eager "to learn and thirst for new experiences, for new sounds, new colours, new concepts of music."[76] Menuhin's fascination with classical Indian music ran deeply. Soon after his early trips to India in 1952 and 1954, Menuhin embarked on a holistic engagement with Indian music in body, mind, and spirit as he enthusiastically performed, studied, and promoted it with Ravi Shankar, Ali Akbar Khan, and Chatur Lal.

As Menuhin embarked on his study and practice of yoga during the 1950s and 1960s, he was also productive in his study of Indian music. He enthusiastically shared his knowledge and understanding of Indian music with the public through articles in newspapers and magazines, and on scripts for TV and radio programs. Some of his efforts "to bring

East and West closer together on a cultural plane" coincided with his classical-music concerts, such as in Sydney, Australia, in 1962.[77] By the time he first released the recording *West Meets East* with Ravi Shankar in 1966, Menuhin had already prepared the detailed program notes.[78] Even as he became absorbed in other projects in the 1970s and 1980s, Menuhin continued to promote Indian music and support the country's cultural events. He helped welcome Indira Gandhi to Great Britain with a message for the India League in 1971, and he wrote a message in 1972 for the Silver Jubilee anniversary celebration of India's independence. Menuhin enthusiastically participated in the BBC's World Phone-In with his reminiscences of India, and he contributed to a Festival of India celebration in the US in 1984.

Menuhin "felt all along the necessity to protect the arts of India,"[79] and he became a special steward of Indian music on his educational mission. As he sought to illuminate the deep cultural connections he found between the West and the East, Menuhin wanted to show how and why Indian music was relevant to the world today. He continually worked out three main ideas about Indian music in his essays and programs. The first idea traces the origins of Western music back to a source in Indian music, the second assesses how Western music adapted to Eastern influences, and the third proposes ways Western music could benefit from exposure to Indian music. Menuhin's efforts to work out these three ideas reflect his passion for Eastern music and his steady zeal to uncover the depths of its meaning in relation to Western music, and I discuss each in more detail below.

INDIAN MUSIC AS A SOURCE FOR WESTERN MUSIC

Menuhin's fascination to uncover the deep cultural connections he sensed between the West and the East, first inspired by his studies with Enesco and later his yoga practice, led him to believe Western music evolved from the East, along with influences from the Middle East, Hungary, Spain, and Africa. Perhaps stemming from his childhood fascination with gypsy music, Menuhin held that the gypsies were the link between East and West as they carried their music from India to Eastern Europe and eventually to Spain where it transformed into flamenco. In short, Eastern Europe became a musical crossroads of cultures from which music evolved in northern Europe and beyond.[80]

Menuhin emphasized this East-West connection in the recording *West Meets East* not only by recording ragas with Shankar but also by including Enesco's "Sonata for Piano and Violin" on the album. To Menuhin, Enesco embodied this link, and Menuhin highlighted how the Romanian composer represented a common cross-cultural connection between himself and Shankar in his program notes to the recording.[81] Menuhin found that Enesco's Sonata "miraculously translated his people's improvised gypsy musical idiom into a formal and complete Western sonata. . . . This could only happen through the mind and heart of one born and bred of a union between the intuitive world of the East and the crystallized and consolidated world of the West."[82]

Menuhin finally was able to formally communicate his idea about East-West musical connections on a program titled "From the Sitar to the Guitar" in 1995. Working with Ravi Shankar on this program from Brussels, Menuhin proposed his plan "to illustrate the relationship between classical Indian music and Spanish Flamenco through the Gypsies who came from India."[83] Shankar enthusiastically supported Menuhin's idea and agreed to participate. He praised Menuhin's vision: "Who but you in the West would have such a magnanimous heart and love for other traditions of art and culture to do this!"[84] The program showed "the great trek of the Gypsies—the Romanians—from India to Spain both North and South of the Mediterranean over a thousand years," which gave Menuhin "the realization of a lifetime desire to illustrate and make heard the voices of the oppressed."[85]

Still a spokesman and advocate of Indian music in the last years of his life, Menuhin reiterated his pet theory in a book review on Indian music in 1997. While he commended the work to be balanced and objective, Menuhin reflected more on the greatness of Ravi Shankar and world music. He wished the book had said more about "the great linking thread between India and Spain that connects the musical nomads of Rajasthan via the Gypsies to the music of Andalusia."[86]

How Western Music Adapted to Eastern Influences

As Menuhin developed his idea of cross-fertilization between music of the East and West, he simultaneously explored how Western music adapted to the influences of Indian music. He often compared and contrasted the two musics in his articles and programs, and he deduced that Western music reflected a culture of compromise resulting from a stream of myriad influences. Such compromises, Menuhin thought, yielded Western music's tuning system of equal temperament and its approach to time and harmonic closure. He found Western music to be "contrary to the very spirit of Indian classical music which is timeless and which shuns the clear and pronounced start or finish," while he believed Western harmony caused restrictions of "certain freedoms, elaborations, ornamentations, conventions and cadenzas of private initiation which exist in Indian music until this day."[87]

Menuhin particularly thought Western harmony constricted free improvisation and ornamentation as it adapted to influences from Indian music. To him, the pure and sacred Indian music represented a synthesis of art and science, with its freedom in improvisation and its rhythmic and melodic structure in the ragas. Yet Menuhin advocated for a meeting of the two cultures in the spirit of diversity: "Western music has a long history of absorbing and appropriating other influences. . . . It thus becomes apparent that this meeting of opposites . . . is merely one more such fruitful encounter in a long history of such nuptial flights."[88]

Through his articles and programs, Menuhin communicated his ideas about how Western music adapted to Eastern influences to the educated layperson. He typically introduced the sitar, which was an exotic and foreign instrument to most readers and audiences, and he tried to frame the sounds of Indian music within known contexts of Western music. For example, he liked to explain how certain melodic strands in Western music adapted Indian melodic ideas that had also evolved into Greek, Gypsy, and Arabic scales and modes. He framed the standard Western musical elements of rhythm, instrumentation, and form in terms of the Indian raga and art of improvisation. In particular, Menuhin opened the door to American listeners through the key rhythmic element of Indian music by relating it to jazz rhythm. Menuhin also provided a Western analog for Indian melody by comparing the raga to the twelve-tone row, which he found to be "the equivalent of the Indian raga or model scale," although "the [twelve-tone] system has not yet discovered the subtleties and varieties of mood which come of using a limited number—nine, eight or seven tones—as the Indian musician knows so well."[89]

Beyond comparing such musical elements between West and East, Menuhin believed sharing his knowledge of Indian music would help open people's minds. His unwavering belief in unity in diversity always appealed to the higher aspects of the human spirit: "Despite the vast contrast in civilizations, the wonderful thing about mankind is precisely that we have it within us, instinctively and consciously, to conduct and find a sympathetic response for everything, including our opposites."[90]

How Western Music Could Benefit from Indian Music

Just as Menuhin found the practice of yoga to benefit his violin playing and teaching, he believed a cross-cultural fertilization with Indian music could benefit Western musicians. In particular, Menuhin held that Indian musicians were especially skilled in ornamentation, melody, and rhythm, with an "acute and accurate sense of hearing and pitch," and that we could cross-fertilize without "damaging the roots and trunk of the tree of India . . . yet bring forth wonderful fruit."[91] Menuhin enumerated six areas where Western music could benefit from and be influenced by Indian music, most of which echo yogic spiritual overtones regarding flexibility, freedom, and unity. Menuhin also cites improvisation as a means to unlock the creative spirit in a performer. His list of how Indian music might influence Western music, with yoga-related concepts in bold, includes:

> (1) the **flexibility** of the tone-row; (2) melodic **freedom** and invention, including ornamentation; (3) the peculiar Indian genius for **uniting** melody and beat, [which he claims is] so different from the African genius as developed in American jazz; (4) the ability to improvise, together with the particular training required and the **release** of inspired creative energies in the performer; (5) the quality of serenity, a type of unique, exalted and personal **expression of union with the infinite**, as in infinite love; (6) the study of the incredibly complex rhythmic organization of Indian music. . . . This is a prime example of unbounded intellectual complexity holding the emotional surge in check."[92]

Menuhin believed Western violinists in particular had much to learn from Indian violinists, especially by studying Indian techniques like the glissando: "Our music and our stance is, in fact, alien to the perfection of the glissando technique as it exists in Indian music."[93] Menuhin also admired how Indian musicians have great accuracy of pitch and ability to play in tune "unencumbered by the fuzz of the keyboard harmonies."[94]

Menuhin further suggested ways Indian music could revitalize Western contemporary composers by providing new compositional resources. While he did not fault modern composers, who he thought have lost the quality of "serene exaltation" he found in Indian music since Western civilization has little of that quality to draw on, he issued a kind of call to action for them to "help us find this quality again."[95]

Through print, television, and musical recordings, Menuhin shared his knowledge of Indian music, which he found to be an "unbelievably rich and wonderfully inspiring culture."[96] Ever the idealist, Menuhin believed the cultural exchange between Indian and Western cultures benefited not only musicians but Westerners in general, helping to acquire such values as non-commercialism, a new sense of time, and order of life. He sought to help people understand "this incredible contrast between the American and the Indian, between the new world and that very old world of India and when we will be given a chance to deepen our understanding of each other and to share the future in harmony and inspiration."[97]

Chapter 5

Yoga Path of Devotion

Menuhin's Philosophical and Spiritual Beliefs

In addition to demonstrating the paths of the Yoga of Action in the body (*karmayoga*) and the Yoga of Knowledge in the mind (*jñanayoga*), Menuhin's selfless service to humanity and views on the spiritual concept of "Oneness" align with the path of the Yoga of Devotion, or *bhaktiyoga*. Although proudly Jewish, Menuhin didn't attend synagogue. Rather, he embraced such core yoga spiritual values as *isvarapranidhana* (devotion to a Higher Power), *karuna* (compassion), *ahimsa* (non-harming), *aparigraha* (non-greed), *dhyana* (meditation), and *samadhi* (absorption). Throughout his life, Menuhin demonstrated a strong commitment to making the world a better place, and he consistently expressed his compassion for humanity, especially for the voiceless and underserved. He framed this compassion within his devotion to a Higher Power, and he worked to remove obstacles to world peace and to promote cultural unity. These principles, which go back to early periods before he encountered yoga but which also remained strong as he integrated the practice into his life, demonstrate Menuhin's commitment to some of yoga's most important values, including being a force for good in the world and the concept of unity in all life.

Two areas of Menuhin's life especially demonstrate important aspects of yogic teachings and practice in the spiritual realm. One area is his long-term humanitarian service, including his extensive commitment to numerous music-related educational and community programs and his notable involvement in some of the world's most important humanitarian and public service organizations. The other area is his philosophical/

spiritual belief system, which he outlined in essays and articles and which included his embrace of Indian music. One of his most notable writings that mirrors his long embrace of spirituality in yoga is his "My Prayer."

Humanitarian Service

Menuhin's humanitarian service may productively be viewed and interpreted through the lens of yoga most broadly in the way it aligns with the first limb of *yamas* (universal moral injunctions). As outlined in the first limb of yoga, the principles of *ahimsa* (nonviolence, harmlessness), *satya* (truthfulness), *asteya* (non-stealing), *brahmacarya* (chastity, religious studentship), and *aparigrahah* (renunciation of unnecessary belongings) involve a spiritual responsibility of citizenship in the world. In his life's work, Menuhin consistently embraced the belief of his guru Iyengar that the fruits of one's actions should be dedicated to the Lord or to humanity.[1] Menuhin's belief that music could be a powerful force for healing and goodness in the world reflects this core tenet of yoga philosophy, and it is particularly evident in two notable areas of his life: music-related programs to serve the community and his leadership roles in world organizations.

MUSIC-RELATED PROGRAMS TO SERVE THE COMMUNITY

One of Menuhin's most lasting contributions to music and humanity was his longstanding commitment to community initiatives. Among the initiatives he spearheaded were Live Music Now (LMN), the Mozart Fund, MUS-E: Music in Europe, the International Yehudi Menuhin Foundation (IYMF), and the Assemblée de cultures européennes (ACE, or Assembly of European Cultures). Each initiative points to the ways in which Menuhin's life may be understood as manifestations of the yogic principles that he explored with Iyengar and absorbed through his yoga practice.

Of all Menuhin's community initiatives, LMN is perhaps the strongest example of how he applied the yogic principles of service and devotion by using the power of music to provide spiritual comfort to those in need. Created in 1977 by Menuhin and Ian Stoutzker, and still in existence today, LMN grew from the seed of an idea the composer Peggy Glanville-Hicks told Menuhin during the war years.[2] Glanville-Hicks had envisioned a project that would equally benefit struggling young artists and the public who could not, or would not, go to concerts. Menuhin built on her service idea, reinforced by his own experiences performing for Allied troops during World War II and sparked by an experience of Diana Menuhin, who saw a needy violin student playing for money in the London tube. The organization LMN coupled Menuhin's educational and humanitarian missions. It partnered with and trained young professional musicians to perform in community spaces throughout the UK, ranging from hospitals to hospices and from prisons to schools. Menuhin's vision for the organization states both its musical and social purpose and captures his strong belief in the power of music: "Music, amongst all the great arts, is the language which penetrates most deeply into the human spirit, reaching people through every barrier, disability, language and circumstance. This is why it has been my dream to bring music back into the lives of those people whose lives are especially prone to stress and suffering . . . so that it might comfort, heal and bring delight."[3]

Menuhin launched another humanitarian project named the Mozart Fund in 1990, one year before the commemoration of the bicentennial of Mozart's death. He wanted to raise funds for worthy causes by levying a royalty on performances of Mozart's music, which he knew would abound in 1991. Menuhin specifically sought to help organizations that worked to avert catastrophes like famine, disease, pollution, explosions of social or racial violence, and war. While he acknowledged the crucial work of relief organizations such as the Red Cross, his idea was to support organizations that help prevent disasters. The project first gained traction in Switzerland in 1991 with organizations including the Bellerive Foundation to save the Alps from environmental damage, the Swiss Committee for the Prevention of Torture, and the Order of Malta to fight leprosy.[4] Even though the European Parliament ratified legislation to support the initiative eleven years later, Menuhin's idea was never fully implemented. Sadly, it seems to have faded away.

Menuhin developed other important initiatives in the 1990s that apply yogic philosophical principles of service to humanity, including MUS-E: Music in Europe.[5] Launched in Brussels in 1994, the program targeted schools in underserved neighborhoods, most of which had a multiracial student population. Menuhin wanted to help circumvent racial prejudice and intolerance while supporting the children's creative, emotional, and intellectual development. In keeping with his holistic belief system, Menuhin ensured that yoga would have a strong presence in the school by offering yoga classes to the older children, along with classes in tai chi and martial arts. The cross-cultural program, which first took root in the

European cities of Brussels, Paris, London, Berlin, Bern, and Budapest, also introduced singing, mime, acting, and dance for younger children.[6]

In the 1990s, Menuhin's international fame and stature enabled him to raise funds for his humanitarian causes. He created the International Yehudi Menuhin Foundation (IYMF) in 1991 as an umbrella organization for his projects and as a means to channel European Community funds. Established by royal decree in Brussels, the IYMF furthered the missions of the Yehudi Menuhin School, the Gstaad Academy, the European String Teachers Association, LMN, and MUS-E. The IYMF still exists today to serve Menuhin's "humanist dream of giving a voice to the voiceless through the arts, irrespective of background, and building a civilization of reciprocity."[7]

Two years before his death, Menuhin devoted himself to ACE, a cultural forum that advocates for underrepresented or stateless groups, such as the Roma and the Basque. Menuhin believed, based on his early-life lessons in "unity in diversity" and now the yogic principle of service, that Europe "could only be understood via the diversity of its cultures . . . they should be given a platform where they can express their hopes and responsibilities and bring their contribution to the European Union."[8] Menuhin presided over ACE's first meeting, held under the auspices of the European Parliament in Brussels in November 1997 and attended by delegates from fifty cultural minorities.

LEADERSHIP ROLES IN WORLD ORGANIZATIONS

Menuhin's commitment to serving world organizations in leadership roles also reflects his yogic imperative to put the fruits of one's actions into serving humanity. Through the responsibility he felt to public service more generally, Menuhin especially embodied the yogic principles of non-harming, compassion, and devotion as he assumed important leadership positions to promote causes like cultural unity and world peace. He also channeled his seemingly limitless capacity for compassion to help organizations advocating for animal rights, like the Puffin Club, and human rights, like Amnesty International.

Beginning in the mid-1950s, when his yoga study and practice with Iyengar began to take root, Menuhin leveraged his stature as a world-renowned violinist to exert a positive influence on international political discourse. In 1956 he assumed his first two leadership roles in organizations where he could make an impact for humanitarian gains—as president of the Arts Federation of South Africa and as president of the Asian Music

Circle. He tried to further the mission of the South African organization "to encourage opportunities for non-whites to experience and enjoy all the arts"[9] by taking a stand against apartheid. Menuhin kept his vow never to return until the government banished such discrimination, and he finally returned to South Africa in 1995 to conduct Handel's *Messiah*. The Asian Music Circle, a nonprofit organization formed in London in 1953, sought to promote the music, dance, and culture of Asia to a wider audience in Western countries. Menuhin's role as president contributed to the organization's mission, as he helped open doors for Iyengar to give demonstrations and classes in London in the 1950s and 1960s.

From 1969 to 1975, Menuhin's association with the International Music Council (IMC), an autonomous offshoot of UNESCO, provided a bigger platform for his humanitarian work. He especially demonstrated the first yoga *yama* of *ahimsa* in his six-year tenure as president of the IMC by promoting peace between warring political factions. His speeches in Moscow in 1971 and in Toronto in 1975 exemplified his dedication to social justice as he sought to alleviate persecution through his influence. In his Moscow speech, Menuhin spoke out against the restrictions of cultural freedom in the Soviet Union and promoted music as the language of peace. His speech inspired one reporter to write, "Yehudi Menuhin is known throughout the world as an altruist and peacemaker. If each of us adopts his Planetary Philosophy, limitless inner and outer peace can result."[10]

In the September 1975 Toronto convention, Menuhin demonstrated how yogic principles of non-harming and compassion operated in his humanitarian work as he diplomatically weathered a political dilemma between the Arab and Israeli musicians in attendance. That year, UNESCO had censured Israel for not granting cultural autonomy to Arabs in the occupied West Bank. In turn, Israeli delegates of the IMC brought with them a statement rejecting the UN's condemnation of Israel. In what must have been an impassioned opening address to the convention, Menuhin pleaded for tolerance and to separate the cultural mission of the organization from politics: "Never forget we are not here as national delegates *only* representing political state, but as musicians representing humanity's cultures."[11] Menuhin's belief in the power of music as a force for good, and his call for all musicians of the world to transcend their differences, promoted harmony between the Arab and Israeli participants. At the end of the conference the Israeli delegates retracted their statement.

Such yogic principles of compassion and devotion continued to operate throughout Menuhin's life. In the early 1990s, he experienced two highlights in the role of an elder public statesman advocating for humanitarian causes. One was his receipt of Israel's prestigious Wolf Prize in May 1991. Upon receiving this honor, Menuhin was entitled to address the Knesset, Israel's legislative branch, in Jerusalem. As in Moscow twenty years earlier, he combined diplomacy with his humanitarian duty. In his speech, Menuhin first established his credentials as a Jew who was a descendant of the Hassidic rabbinical sect and linked to the international Jewish community through his musical career. Then he spoke about the current state of political affairs in Israel. He described his vision for true unity in the country, in which he hoped for "an eventual confederation, on the Swiss model of neighboring cultures, with Jerusalem becoming a shared capital."[12] True to his compassionate vision and principles, Menuhin also visited communities in East Jerusalem and on the West Bank, where he saw "sufficient evidence of an unacceptable ruthlessness on the part of the occupying Israeli forces to make me feel, as a Jew, utterly appalled."[13] The day after his speech in the Knesset, Menuhin met with King Hussein in Jordan and was moved by his "heartfelt words when he said that his dearest and greatest dream was for a Semitic federation of peoples."[14] In keeping with his principles of compassion and selfless service, Menuhin donated his Wolf Prize money to various Israeli organizations dedicated to the legal protection and support of Palestinians and their children's education. As the ongoing discord between Arabs and Israelis continues nearly thirty years later, Menuhin's compassionate actions model service-oriented pathways toward reconciliation today.

Menuhin's second public-life highlight occurred in 1992. That year, UNESCO named him an ambassador of goodwill. Menuhin conducted the gala concert in San Francisco for the fiftieth anniversary celebration of the founding of the UN—an especially meaningful milestone since he had performed at a concert inaugurating the UN charter back in 1942. Menuhin made a speech during the celebration in which he "chided the rich nations of the world for denying the UN their support, called on the USA and the UK to rejoin UNESCO, and pleaded for a 'global conscience' towards the world's trouble."[15] Members of the audience, which included Lech Walesa of Poland and Princess Margaret of the UK, rose to their feet at the end, and Menuhin felt gratified by the ovation as it symbolized "a fundamental commitment to internationalism and peace."[16]

Menuhin used his international platform to advance his humanitarian causes as he met with diplomats, politicians, business leaders, economists, and others who directly influenced people's lives. He wanted to learn from such leaders but also hoped that "occasionally perhaps they may lend me their ears reciprocally, how best to advance the causes, cultural and humanitarian, that are dear to my heart."[17] While most of Menuhin's numerous lectures and speeches convey his deep compassion for humanity and strong advocacy for cultural unity, some of them point specifically to his engagement with yogic beliefs and values. For example, in 1969, the year Menuhin assumed the presidency of the IMC, he delivered two notable speeches. In one titled "Creative Attitude" given at the US Embassy in Paris on March 3, Menuhin seized the opportunity to speak about spiritual concerns as well as economic, political, diplomatic, and military issues. With confidence and boldness that showed no fear or trepidation about addressing such heads of state as Presidents Richard Nixon of the US and Charles de Gaulle of France, Menuhin framed his message for how truth and beauty might heal the divisive and destructive forces in the world within a universal sense of a spiritual force. In keeping with his own belief in Oneness, he called on the healing power of a universal life force, like the yogic concept of *isvara*. He noted how the Western monotheistic view of absolutism is "tearing at the very seams of society. It is quite one thing to conceive of a unity to which you belong: it is quite another to conceive of yourself as the fountainhead, the *raison d'etre* of that unity. This is the fatal flaw, deriving from stupidity and vanity, which has twisted mankind's monotheism into mankind's megalomania."[18]

In another 1969 speech titled "Heaven on Earth" given at the Royal Commonwealth Hall to the Conservation Society, an organization in which he also served as president, Menuhin took up the banner of preserving the world's natural environment. As he expounded on how humans must be the earth's custodians and bring the infinite variety of life into harmony, he referenced the phenomenon of vibrations, an important yogic concept about sound and its power to communicate. He framed vibrations of higher sense perception like a yogic power, which the artist must call upon to create and conserve beauty: "As a musician, I live with vibrations, a state which is neither animate nor inanimate, but is common to both. Vibrations are of all phenomena the ones which allow us to touch, as it were, the most distant source, both in space and time. Because we are vibrating, pulsating beings, we can sense and in fact relive the sensations, sentiments, impulses and thoughts of thousands of other musicians, and as musicians we can communicate these to millions of people."[19]

In the last two decades of his life, Menuhin continued to deliver speeches to plead for support of music that also resonated with yogic principles of spiritual freedom. His capacity for helping others, and for being of service to humanity, impacted a host of musical, social, and environmental organizations, including the 1980 World Music Day, the Princess Alice Hospice, and Compassion in World Farming. Perhaps most poignantly, after his installation in the House of Lords in January 1994, Menuhin advocated for how the power of music "enables us to breathe and to dream. For Man acts and behaves according to his visions, be they ideals or simply ambitions. It is these dreams which shape our lives."[20]

Philosophy and Spiritual Beliefs

In addition to his humanitarian work, Menuhin developed a number of powerful spiritual and philosophical ideas that reflect larger yogic principles of devotion. Highlights of Menuhin's philosophy are captured beautifully in the "Yehudi Menuhin Philosophenweg" ("Yehudi Menuhin Philosophy Path"), a walking path between Gstaad and Saanen with stations to reflect on twelve Menuhin quotes.[21] While some of these ideas were likely influenced by his childhood mentors and Jewish upbringing, others clearly drew upon his yoga practice and readings in Eastern philosophies as an adult. Many of his writings, including essays, articles, and lectures, reflect his fervent spiritual devotion and deep compassion for the human race, but his approach to spirituality and philosophy is also evident in his explorations of Indian music as well as in a prayer document that he worked on during the last decade of his life.

As the key concept in yoga is "union," Menuhin's belief system embraced unity and what he called Oneness of a universal life force. Menuhin's mastery of body and mind produced a positive, unified stream of creativity flowing into and out of this divine life force, similar to the work of a yogi. Through being part of this unified stream in music, Menuhin found his own version of *kaivalya* (absolute spiritual freedom). His philosophy incorporated many other underlying yogic concepts and principles, which in turn extended to music itself. Indian music especially encapsulated Menuhin's spiritual principles. In the final analysis, music and yoga provided Menuhin with a means to the same end: spiritual oneness and wholeness with all of creation.

Menuhin traces his attraction to Indian thought to his own ancestral roots in the East: "My conviction that the farther I travelled east, the closer I came to my origins guaranteed I should find India the primal ocean whose waters flowing westward across the centuries fed my familiar streams of ideas, attitude, and music."[22] His contact with Eastern culture and ideas colored not only some of Menuhin's most important musical achievements but also his entire belief system. His philosophical and spiritual writings eschew Western independence for Eastern concepts of unity, and he valued community over the individual. Some aspects of Menuhin's belief system echo Hindu concepts of reincarnation and *karma* (action, work, deed; universal law of cause and effect) as he pondered life's problems and dualities. For example, he believed that our "multiple lives" cycle through our selfish pursuits and lack of vision for the future as "we ruthlessly forge our power . . . because we only live once, which I personally do not believe."[23]

Menuhin points to the German Jewish philosopher Constantin Brunner (1862–1937), whose work he first came to know in 1938, as another strong influence in his belief system. Menuhin thought Brunner's ideas prepared him for his encounter with yogic teachings since the philosopher had also studied Hinduism.[24] Menuhin must have absorbed Brunner's ideas on the unity of all spiritual disciplines as he developed his own concept of Oneness. As a service to this "spiritual mentor," Menuhin served on the board of the International Constantin Brunner Institute (ICBI) in the Hague until his death.[25]

While to my knowledge Menuhin never claimed to be a theosophist, one cannot help but make associations between that philosophy and his own beliefs. On the scribbled notes for his "Music and Religion" lecture at Kings College in 1991, Menuhin made one intriguing reference: "Theocracy—all is holy."[26] After he delivered the lecture, Menuhin responded to a request from the dean of King's College to summarize his talking points and to send his concluding prayer, but he did not mention the point about theocracy in his typed letter.[27] Yet since he noted it in his handwritten outline so prominently, he probably mentioned it in his talk. Certainly Menuhin's belief system resonates with the theosophist's "open-minded inquiry into world religions, philosophy, science, and the arts in order to understand the wisdom of the ages, respect the unity of all life, and help people explore spiritual self-transformation."[28]

MENUHIN'S PAPERS, LECTURES, AND OTHER WRITINGS: 1951–1999

Menuhin expressed his spiritual and philosophical beliefs in an abundance of papers, lectures, and articles throughout his adult life. The breadth and depth of his writing demonstrates how far his engagement with yoga and the teachings of his guru Iyengar influenced his basic thinking about existence, art, and the creative human spirit.[29] While his astounding output of writings and lectures covers a broad array of themes and topics, I will point to some key examples that reflect how deeply yoga impacted his spiritual and philosophical belief system over time.

As early as 1951, just after he first encountered yoga, Menuhin delivered a speech to a group that advocated for a new world federal government in Australia. In this speech, he articulated his developing belief about the continuity of the spirit and even embraced reincarnation. He called for a new faith to be established in great humility, in which all people and races are "born of the same inspired vision of oneness and justice and they represent merely various stages and aspects of life and man's progressive emancipation and slow maturation."[30] Later in the 1950s in a speech titled "Art and Science as Related Concepts" given to the Royal Institution of Great Britain, Menuhin described intuition in yoga-like terms as "the awareness of eternity and infinity, of duality within the unity, of the cycle of life, of matter and of all occurrence."[31]

In a 1967 lecture at St. Andrews University titled "Is an Unspiritual Education Possible?" Menuhin continued to expound on his ideas about the continuity and momentum of spiritual forces at work in education using terms that invoke yogic concepts like *asmita* (ego, or I-ness), *atma* (soul), and *karma*. He expressed his core belief that "the spiritual is inherent to and inalienable from all men [within] the conception of an infinite I-consciousness [and] a Great Being of all time," even as a fusion of choice, free-will, and self-determination results from the "experience of cause and effect and a degree of compulsion."[32]

As Menuhin sought to inspire hope for humanity with his positivist ideas, his words affirmed yogic principles of spiritual unity in the work of artists. For example, in his 1973 address "How Does the Creative Artist Express the Spirit of His Time?" delivered at the Dean of Windsor's Symposium at St. George's Chapel at Windsor Castle, England, he said, "I am convinced that life is not propelled by, but attracted to order, balance and understanding; stated in the words of the soul, it is harmony, wisdom and compassion."[33] He further called for the artist to widen the spiritual domain of humanity by preparing people to awake from our living dream-state to the full "mystical union" state of wakefulness beyond our life. A year later in his lecture "Creativity," given to the Smithsonian Resident Associate Program in 1974, Menuhin invoked more yogic concepts about removing obstacles that block one's true self from shining forth. He described how creativity was a birthright of every living creature, but it is "covered up by pain, anxiety, fear, and mistrust."[34] Menuhin's view of creativity also suggests yogic concepts of one-pointed attention, equanimity, awareness, and union as he defined it as "a state of grace, a state of being in which everything converges, in which time and space are focused into one point . . . that balanced condition that considers our past heritage, present state, and projection of the future . . . a state of heightened awareness [of the] human condition when the personal and the universal merge."[35]

Yogic concepts continue to reverberate in Menuhin's later speeches. In his 1982 talk "A Recognition of Art as Hope," given at the Royal Scottish Museum in Edinburgh, Menuhin called on the artist to channel the gifts from the Divine. He also connected the physical and spiritual realms in a way that echoes Iyengar's belief that what we first practice and absorb through the body penetrates the deeper levels of mind and spirit: "I firmly believe that ethical and aesthetical values and truths derive from, or are parallel to, or are a mirror of, physical facts."[36] His message to the Conference on Music, Mathematics, and Mysticism in 1985 touched on spiritual ideas that reflect yogic concepts of unity, consciousness, and removing ignorance: "Life is a never-ending discovery of unity of all creation. Like all discoveries it follows upon an awareness, an intuitive sense of beings to a greater plan or power, a greater creation, whether we call that greater power God or consciousness or whatever, it is to this reality that we address our inner vision. We try to close the infinite gap of our ignorance."[37] In his 1987 talk "Tolerance," given to the King's College in London, Menuhin emphasized how education must replace ignorance, the root of all obstacles in yogic philosophy, and how compassion must replace judgment of others. He reaffirmed his core belief of the interconnectedness within all creation with a Brunner quote that further substantiates this Hindu belief: "Everything is alive, or conscious, or possessed of the latent capacity for life and consciousness; there is a hint of the divine spirit in every atom."[38]

Menuhin published a number of significant articles that capture how deeply yogic values influenced his spiritual and philosophical thinking in the last two decades of his life. In his 1980 lecture "Man: By Definition a Religious Animal: Of the Sacredness of Consciousness, Conscience and Choice," which was printed the next year,[39] Menuhin viewed all deities as manifestations of One, like the yogic understanding of *isvara*, and he sought a common Higher Power that exists through all names for God. His twenty-page typed essay "On Oneness," which appeared in two parts in *The Times* (London) in August 1989 as "Escape the Fate of the Dinosaur" and "Pray for an Orphaned Race,"[40] echoes the yogic principle of union and unity of spirit.

In the last decade of his life, Menuhin continued to deliver lectures and write essays that reflect how his spiritual beliefs and philosophy parallel yogic principles. Like the yogic principle of removing the veil of *avidya* (ignorance) to see the true self, Menuhin challenges human beings to uncover the layer of ignorance through creative discovery in his 1993 unpublished essay "Human Creativity": "What we call discovery is only the revelation of a previous ignorance, as the discovery of America or the law of gravity by Galileo, or the perfect fifth, the basic musical interval by Pythagoras, or of Einstein's equation between matter and energy, and the transformation of either one into the other."[41] His 1994 article titled "Some Ephemeral Thoughts on Tolerance and Peace For Madame Lalumiere," which was also translated into French, reiterates much of his earlier philosophy of harmony and unity but set up within the yogic value of equilibrium and equanimity: "Understanding the shifting bounds of tolerance is essential to understanding the ever-changing harmonies and dissonances which mark the dynamic character of peace. Both have an inner and an outer aspect—centrifugal and centripetal. Both the forces of rejection (of repulsion) and the forces of attraction are in equilibrium over a shorter or longer period of carrying intensity, and each reflects the inner to the outer and back."[42]

MENUHIN'S FOUR PHILOSOPHICAL/SPIRITUAL THEMES

From a survey of Menuhin's many papers, lectures, and articles, four important recurring themes pertaining to his transcendental philosophical and spiritual beliefs emerge, all of which may be interpreted though the lens of yogic teaching and philosophy. The first, and perhaps the most central, is Menuhin's idea about Oneness. As *isvara* signifies the Lord called by many names in yoga philosophy, Menuhin's theme of Oneness holds that all world deities reflect the same essential Divine Spirit and that all life is unified by this life force. A second theme Menuhin returns to throughout his papers is the duality of consciousness, like the yogic concept of the duality between the observer and the observed. A third continually recurring theme, that artists channel the Divine Spirit and so have the opportunity to lift up and even enlighten their fellow human beings, exemplifies Iyengar's teaching that a yogi is responsible for carrying the fruits of their practice, that is, the calm mind, out into the world for the benefit of humankind. Menuhin's fourth important theme relates to the meaning of life itself, as he echoes many of the yogic universal vows and individual practices set forth in the *yamas* and the *niyamas*. I will discuss these four yoga-centered themes in more detail and demonstrate how Menuhin integrated them into his philosophical/spiritual belief system.

Oneness

Menuhin's ideas about Oneness stem from his broad spiritual beliefs that transcended any one religion or dogma, in keeping with his guru's belief that "yoga, like God, is one . . . but people call Him by different names."[43] Like a true citizen of the world, he embraced a "greater power" beyond all its manifestations and a "universal principle of eternal change" that implies "the oneness of the basic material and the one power."[44] He believed Jesus best represents human suffering, compassion, and capacity for love, yet he also revered Lord Buddha, Allah, and Jehovah as the God of Moses and Abraham. For him, faith broke the narrow boundaries of ideology.

As he deepened his unity in diversity belief from earlier years, Menuhin worked out his idea of Oneness to find spiritual unity in his later years. He even admitted that his "On Oneness" theme had become a "continued obsession."[45] Menuhin called for awareness of the deep divisions in humanity's thinking and the willingness to fight over them—a call we could continue to heed today. These divisions, coupled with a "willful selfishness toward the natural world," will only cause us to "await the destiny of the dinosaur."[46] Menuhin also called for a more objective, scientific approach to find the common underlying Higher Power and to transcend the differences and dualities created by the world's three monotheistic religions—Judaism, Christianity, and Islam. Just as science gives humanity a common denominator for polarizations of action and reaction, matter and energy, the organic and inorganic, Menuhin viewed God, or the Universe, as one entity and the "mathematics of the Universe constitute one truth."[47]

Just as yoga teaches that the human dilemma is rooted in how the mind blocks the realization of the true self, Menuhin believed that separation from union with all life is the root of humanity's problems and has made us into "spiritual orphans." Reframing the yogic belief that ignorance covers the *atman*, our true nature, and that all life is connected in one creative field (*prakrti*), Menuhin sounds the alarm that we are out of balance. This state of "disequilibrium" results from conflicting views of "normalcy" in physical, spiritual, and intellectual matters, and he advocated for the same yogic ideals of balance and equilibrium.[48]

In his unwavering idealism, Menuhin thought the impulse to believe in a Higher Power lies at the core of the human spirit. We all yearn to be a part of creation, a part of the whole infinite and eternal One. Yet without upholding a common, holistic belief, generating a healing force in the world is almost impossible. Menuhin's solution to achieving the needed union of wholeness with the entire stream of creation was to surrender the ego to that creative force, like *isvarapranidhana*, in order to make room for rebirth.

As Menuhin works out his Oneness idea in such essays as "Man: By Definition a Religious Animal," he touches on the Eastern concept of life cycles and the destruction-creation principle, where death is also the beginning of a new incarnation as symbolized by the Hindu god Shiva. Menuhin called for people to move beyond the warring factions of mono-theistic religions and embrace a higher, universal order of life connected to creation itself and then to assume responsibility for its care. In this idea, Menuhin links an imperative to restore our connection to the Divine Spirit with his core "On Oneness" idea. To achieve such Oneness requires an act of devotion, and Menuhin called for interfaith understanding and reconciliation: "Let us then worship Him, life, ourselves, this God for whom we have many symbols. . . . We must believe and have faith in the one God who is the very essence of life itself, who cannot be separated from us, or put on an altar, except symbolically and is wholly embodied in the Universe and its creatures which in Him and with Him and through Him constitute Him."[49]

Duality of Consciousness

Though less polished than his ideas in "On Oneness," Menuhin's second theme deals with concepts of consciousness and dualities that also relate directly to yoga philosophy. For example, he defines consciousness in terms of a duality between "two intertwined, indissoluble strands, one the *observed*, the other the *observer* that constitute all matter in tangible and intangible ways"[50] (italics mine). Likewise, yoga philosophy sets up consciousness (*citta*) as the duality between the observed (*prakriti*, or the observable field) and the observer (*purusha/atma*, or the seer). Menuhin further defined the transient "observed" and the eternal "observer" in yoga-like terms, where the former includes all tangible organic and inorganic life, matter, and energy that is perceived in the present time (like *prakriti*), and the latter includes all that moves beyond the immediate present (like *purusha*).

Menuhin further framed his two strands of consciousness in dualistic terms between the two pillars of wisdom in the eternal observer and compassion in the transient observed. Like the yogic belief of how ignorance of the true self causes confusion of the observer and the observed, and so leads to our constantly fluctuating consciousness, Menuhin also claimed our power of choice is part of consciousness. As we have seen, he made the case for how our separation from union with all life is the root of humanity's problems and how we must choose to surrender to a Higher Power to join together.

Furthermore, Menuhin posited a duality within the life force itself, as a power beyond us yet also within us. In the moment of human experience, the two strands of consciousness "combine with passion to fire the pulse beating within us that reflects the moment" in a "harmonious vibration in unison."[51] Here, Menuhin embraces such yogic concepts of a *samadhi*-like "timeless moment" as we perceive and gather right knowledge (*pramana*) that results in a spiritual transformation (*parinama*).

The Artist as a Channel of the Divine Spirit

The third central idea in Menuhin's belief system—that when creativity flows unhindered by ignorance and self-centered fear it can channel the Divine Spirit—embodies the principle of what his guru Iyengar believed to be the fruits of yoga: "Here all impressions and afflictions are washed away forever; the consciousness is freed from all flaws to flow clean and clear, for the stream of wisdom and virtue to pour like torrential rain."[52] Menuhin thought artists in this state of creativity have the capacity, and even responsibility, to affect a powerful force for good in the world, just as yogis are responsible for carrying the fruits of their practice out into the world to help humankind. Menuhin believed that through their creations artists could communicate with and influence a wide body of people, who in turn could recognize something in their own selves in this pure communication of human thought and emotion, thereby "releasing them in harmony."[53] Like the ideal of a yogi is to remove the veil of ignorance and all hindrances to the true self, Menuhin believed this state of pure creativity to be the ideal of the artist. He considered humility and acceptance to be the two hallmarks of such an enlightened creative life based on this true motive. He thought that rather than adding to the burdens of future generations, artists add "to the credit side of life by our own lives, our joy in mankind's unique gifts of observing, recreating and communicating."[54]

Naturally, for Menuhin, music was the most communicative of all the arts and so most able to have a powerful, even transcendent, effect on people's lives. Menuhin thought sound, being disembodied, "brings forth a response in our own vibrating selves" as our ears physically transmit real vibrations and encircle us in the vibrations of the world, and he viewed music as a sacred "organized sound," possessing a "creative and magical quality."[55] As Menuhin believed art and mysticism channeled Oneness, he also advocated for other things that promote harmony between adversaries, such as loving care, smiles, sleep, and meditation along with "poetry, art, ecstasy, religion and creation as the *very* fabric and condition of life."[56]

The Meaning of Life

Menuhin's grappling with the meaning of life itself, the fourth main theme in his belief system, also parallels specific areas of yoga philosophy, especially the universal vows and individual practices defined in the *yamas* and the *niyamas*. While Menuhin acknowledged that the search for meaning produces different and subjective views among people, he challenged everyone to live beyond mere enjoyment and self-promotion, regardless of their fellows. To find meaning in life, Menuhin believed we must set guidelines. In his essay "The Meaning of Life," an undated typescript document probably written in the early 1990s, Menuhin sets forth such guidelines, and his points include universal principles that embrace all three dimensions of the body, mind, and spirit:

1. Strive to make yourself into one who is trusted by all living things through sustaining them.

2. Be helpful, be kind, and give counsel to others.

3. Show interest instead of indifference.

4. Exercise love instead of hate.

5. Learn to be a good trustee of your body, which has been entrusted to your temporary keeping.

6. Share with others all that is beautiful.

7. Revere and follow those living examples who enshrine the spirit within and beyond each of us.

In 1991 Menuhin circulated this theme about the meaning of life in a number of publications. One article in *Life* magazine begins with his affirmation of Oneness and the principle of unity in diversity: "The meaning of life lies in the oneness of all creation, which combines supreme diversity with supreme interdependence."[57] He elaborated on how "we are one with creation in time and space," and he warned how individuals, society, and the whole world now are learning the consequences of actions (*karma*), namely exploiting the planet and people.[58]

That same year, a German publisher in Düsseldorf asked Menuhin for his ideas on this subject, asking him, "What do you understand as the meaning of life?" Menuhin reframed his Oneness idea within his respect for life: "To protect this most glorious mystery of nature, to contribute to the well-being of succeeding generations of life—of all life."[59] Taking a yogic-centered approach, Menuhin warns against separating the union of opposites in human nature, like thought and feeling, emotion and rationality, intuition and reason, since one is the "eternal source of living energy" while the other is "eternity itself—pure mathematics—in all its parts of the whole," and he lays out other opposites that must remain in balance and bound together in yogic union and "forever go in tandem" like yin/yang, day/night, sun/moon, heat/cold, and clarity/darkness.[60]

Perhaps Menuhin's response to a letter from a fifth grader in Massachusetts best captures how his spiritual beliefs were grounded in the yogic perspective of unity. As part of his survey of famous people, the young student asked Menuhin, "Do you believe in God?" Menuhin answered in striking simplicity: "Yes, as part of every smallest crumb of matter organic and inorganic. Through the mystery of our infinite unity."[61]

Indian Music

Indian philosophy, as absorbed by Menuhin in the 1950s through his work with Iyengar and his own studies, would profoundly influence many of Menuhin's ideas about music in general. Most directly, Indian philosophy led to his long-term fascination and interest in Indian music. To Menuhin, Indian music provided the same means to the spiritual end of yoga, that is, spiritual unity and wholeness with all of creation. It resonated strongly with his spiritual beliefs about Oneness and the creative flow of the Divine Spirit through art of all cultures. After his first visit to India in 1952, Menuhin began his own dual process of "absorption and dissolution" of Indian music and culture as he began to understand how India integrates thought, feeling, and imagination "into a complete, however complex, unified whole."[62] For Menuhin, Indian life integrated "the principle of continuity, the stability of an ancient order which allowed for all elements in human existence to find their proper station, their function and their meaning."[63]

In contrast, Menuhin thought Westerners were spiritually fragmented and damaged people who needed to find unity: "Until we, the whole of humanity, can get together again in a divine whole by each contributing our crumb of truth, we shall be condemned forever to the crippled and mutilated civilization we are now only too well acquainted with."[64] He also pointed to essential differences between the Western ideal of individualism and Eastern ideal of oneness as it relates to the arts: "Our classical ballet and in fact all Western art is expressive of personal souls in selfless bodies, whereas Indian art seems to speak of personal bodies in selfless souls."[65]

While he found India's holistic principle of unity to be reflected in the intertwining of its art and culture, Menuhin reflected most deeply on Indian music as a spiritual practice. His astute comparisons between Western and Eastern music resonated with yogic teachings and philosophy: "It [Indian music] is a more contemplative, meditative, and passive form of music. It does not allow the surges of emotion and fury, the interplay of opposing forces to mar its detachment. It invites the listener to attain a state of meditation of oneness, with God."[66]

As Menuhin's belief system integrated concepts he absorbed from yoga philosophy and spirituality and connected them deeply to music, we can see how Indian music in particular embodied the path of the Yoga of Devotion in his life. Menuhin writes of how he found the yogic qualities of unity, healing, and liberation in Indian music's spiritual essence: "As in Indian religion the body and soul have never been divided, so in their music, which is still mainly a votive offering, Indians believe in its therapeutic quality as well as in its spiritual effect . . . Indian music has always stressed the relation of man to the universal and [through its various modes and rhythmic patterns] liberates the higher mind from the limits of physical form."[67]

Menuhin was, after all, a musician first and foremost, and he directed his understanding of Indian music's divine expression to both the player and the listener. In the actual playing of Indian music, and as a violinist himself, Menuhin was especially fascinated by the sarangi, the only bowed stringed instrument traditionally used in India. He reflected on the power of practice and fruits of discipline for players of this instrument: "It takes infinite devotion and patience to master this intricate and complex art to the point where intellectual, emotional and digital control is so completely taken for granted that only the creative impulse can guide and reveal itself."[68] Menuhin points to the devotional essence of Indian music and how the players channeled spiritual qualities in performance. "Remember that in India this music—like all Indian art—is an offering born in the temple; and this temple atmosphere pervades even the concert stage. . . . Thus the Indian musician conjures his music, as it were, out of the void, out of the dimensionless and timeless realm which is the objective of all Hindu philosophical and religious experience."[69]

The listener, too, could achieve a spiritual experience through Indian music. Menuhin describes how Indian music conveys such a spiritual experience, but he could also be describing the yogic concept of *samadhi* (total absorption), communicating "immediacy of experience, the electric instantaneousness which fuses cause and effect," and, as such, expressing "an immediate spiritual and physical state of being together with the moral and physical dedication inherent in the art."[70] Menuhin encouraged listeners to open their ears and hearts to Indian music, meant to "unite us in meditation with the infinite, to produce a hypnotic mood in which we almost leave our physical envelope to join the universal in release and serenity."[71] As listeners witness the rapport between the players in performance, they can understand how "Indian music symbolizes the relationship between man and the mysterious infinity of God. It is the colloquy between a human being and his intimate conscience, an act of faith and abandonment, a self-offering to that which is forever beyond us, as is the mystery within us. It is a dialogue between the melody and the rhythm, between the individual and his fate."[72]

Finally, Menuhin found pure love in Indian music as he viewed yoga and music through the same lens of similar spiritual practices—a state of peace like the yogic concept of *kaivalya* (liberation, or absolute freedom). To him, the music expressed the "Indian quality of serenity, the Indian musician's exalted personal expression of union with the infinite, as in infinite love," and, in this supreme state of liberation, the unblocked creative spirit flowed with divine wisdom and love to allow us to "hear eternity" through the music.[73] In Menuhin's view of Oneness, the inspired and humble musicians who serve as channels for the Divine Spirit ultimately interpret and define what originated from the Divine source. They do not create out of nothingness. Even as they embody wisdom and love, each musician's single voice is "one of an infinite number reflecting the Great Voice," and although this one creative voice partakes in the original creation, it really "renders unto God what is essentially His own."[74]

Menuhin's Prayer and Hopes for Humanity

Menuhin's "My Prayer" captures his spiritual beliefs that echo core principles in the Yoga of Devotion. Written in the last ten years of his life, the prayer exists in slightly different versions dating from 1989 to 1991, including the last six paragraphs in his August 22, 1989, article "Pray for an Orphaned Race" and at the end of his revised 1996 memoir *Unfinished Journey: Twenty Years Later*. The version from Menuhin's typescript synthesizes the four main themes in his belief system—Oneness, consciousness and duality, being a channel of the Divine, and the meaning of life—with universal yogic principles as he prays for good stewardship of all life; unity in all manifestations of creation; the practice of discernment, awareness, and reconciliation of dualities; and seeing God in all deities. As he broadly defines God as "the harmonious coordination of the three cardinal principles of life (a) soul—(b) mind—(c) spirit,"[75] Menuhin offered "My Prayer" as a hope for humankind to transcend the separation from God and to restore unity of soul and spirit. And in keeping with the fifth yoga *niyama, isvarapranidhana*, Menuhin believed the way to achieve this state of wholeness and awareness, or Oneness, was to surrender to a Higher Power.

Menuhin's acts of humanitarian service and expression of his spiritual belief system through his writings demonstrate an important influence of yogic teachings and practice. His actions and words resonate with yogic practice and teaching to remove obstacles that block the true self and surrender to a Higher Power. In his fervor to make the world a better place, the concept of devotion runs throughout his actions and words, along with a search for unity in the dimensions of body, mind, and spirit. Menuhin's practice of music, and his beliefs reflected in his writing about Indian music in particular, provided the path for his spiritual quest. In the end, Menuhin's deep spirituality merged yoga and music into one.

Epilogue

Menuhin's Legacy

Like many people today, Menuhin came to yoga to help solve his bodily aches and pains. Yet after he started practicing it in 1952, yoga ignited a cause-and-effect dynamic that colored every aspect of his life. Menuhin's yoga practice and study—his search for balance and union in the physical, mental, and spiritual realms—influenced his work as a performing musician, an educator, and a humanitarian. His efforts yielded tangible results from concerts and international festivals to practical guides for violin playing to his loftier contributions toward world peace and harmony. He connected yogic spiritual principles especially to Indian music, where he found essential commonalities across musical cultures and in the creative spirit of Oneness. Menuhin believed music had the power to transform people and the world. He eloquently reflected: "Is it possible to ask too much of music? As a child I saw it as an irresistible force for good, uniting the human race at its universal depths beneath divisions, working that magic which Schiller describes in his 'Ode to Joy' as 'binding together what Custom pulls asunder.'"[1] Menuhin never lost such idealism from his childhood. Rather, he found a way to bring it to fruition in his adult life as he integrated his two disciplines of yoga and music.

As both a great musician and a benevolent spirit, Menuhin was a man ahead of his time when he discovered yoga and Indian culture in the 1950s. His pioneering efforts to introduce Westerners to yoga through B. K. S. Iyengar and to Indian music through Ravi Shankar made a strong impact in the public sphere during his lifetime. He helped open the door for others to follow. Beginning as early as the 1960s, yoga began to spread in the West, world music became a popular genre, and the academy began to embrace the study of non-Western music. Menuhin's holistic approach to life and work was also ahead of his time. While wholesome diet, regular exercise, and mindfulness meditation are commonly recognized in mainstream culture today, Menuhin embraced all these practices through yoga.

When Menuhin embarked on his quest to repair his violin technique, he had to first study the obstacles in his body and then go through the painful process of undoing them. He knew "the wrong strength must be let go and a period of 'no strength' endured," and his process "began with the sleep induced by Iyengar."[2] Rather than retreat into privacy to retool his technique, Menuhin remained in the public eye. He applied his yoga lessons mid-career during the 1960s and 1970s, when he was most actively working with Iyengar, as he opened his school in England and advocated for Indian music. Then, in the 1980s and 1990s he used his international platform to promote humanitarian causes and zealously wrote reflective articles and essays pertaining to his belief system. Menuhin summarized the fruits of all his efforts: "My search has been one of the main lines of my life, a stabilizing element, an ongoing effort, a lasting satisfaction. The sureness of childhood has been regained, with added intellectual stiffening . . . I have learned that harsh whips of determination cannot drive one to performing pitch, but that one is led there by the quiet exercise of principles grasped by the mind and absorbed by the body over stubborn years of faith."[3]

Like a yogi who applies *asana* practice to deeper levels of human understanding, Menuhin integrated his musical lessons learned from yoga into life: "I have understood that no experience can be isolated from violin playing, that the flexibility with which one holds violin and bow, the mastery which does not grab or dominate, has illuminating parallels in human relations."[4] He gratefully passed on his experience to others, feeling "thankful to have been obliged to discover and assimilate so much," and for acquiring "something of value to impart to others."[5] And finally, in his search for both physical and psychological healing, Menuhin found "bliss" in yoga as the "ideal solution" through natural, rather than artificial, means.[6]

Menuhin's Relevance to Our World Today

Why is Menuhin's story still relevant today? Although he was born over a hundred years ago and launched an early and brilliant career that spanned the 1920s to the 1990s, his search for meaning and his spiritual quest resonate in our fast-paced and technology-driven twenty-first century. His work influenced not only the world during his lifetime but our current world, with far-reaching implications as we seek to find answers to life's complex questions.

Menuhin's concerns are still with us today. In many ways they have gotten worse in our polarized society of warring political factions, climate crises, and breakdown of democratic ideals like the common good. Yet Menuhin's ideals for healing still ring true, and younger musicians are carrying on his legacy of integrating spiritual principles and crossing musical boundaries. For example, two classical violinists named Melissa White and Elena Urioste have created the holistic program Intermission,[7] which encourages a union of body, mind, and spirit through music-making, yoga, and meditation.

The impact of the Yehudi Menuhin School also lives on today, not only by continuing to train young violinists but by supporting established violinists like Nicola Benedetti. An alumna of the school and a former student of Boyarsky, Benedetti is now a violin virtuoso and a rising star in the classical music world. At age ten she began to study at the school and at age eleven she performed the Bach Double Concerto for Menuhin. Although Menuhin died when she was just eleven years old, Benedetti's lasting impressions of the maestro are of his kindness and gentleness. She recognized Menuhin's strikingly "calm presence," explaining, "When he walked into the room you could tell something changed."[8] And, like Menuhin, she crosses musical boundaries, such as in her 2016 recording of jazz musician Wynton Marsalis's Violin Concerto with the Philadelphia Orchestra.[9]

The violinist Daniel Hope, son of Menuhin's longtime assistant Eleanor Hope and Christopher Hope, worked closely with Menuhin in his formative years and considers Menuhin to be his "musical grandfather."[10] Hope especially carries on Menuhin's legacy through his continued involvement with Live Music Now and as a musical activist.[11] Hope performed many times under Menuhin's conducting baton, including Menuhin's final concert on March 7, 1999, in Dusseldorf. For an encore that night, Hope dedicated Maurice Ravel's *Kaddisch* to Menuhin, as the elder musician sat among the orchestra players and listened.[12] Hope thinks this encore may have been prophetic. The term "kaddish" typically refers to the Judaic "Mourner's Kaddish" recited at prayer services for the dead, and five days later Menuhin died.[13] Hope's 2016 album *My Tribute to Yehudi Menuhin* pays homage to the great violinist on his centenary. It includes pieces Hope played with Menuhin as a child and other works Menuhin himself championed, like Ravel's moving *Kaddisch*.

Closer to home, a colleague at Emory, Heidi Senungetuk, surprised me during a dinner conversation about my Menuhin and yoga project in February 2022. She told me that Menuhin had made a huge impact on her as a young violin student growing up in Alaska. Now an ethnomusicologist as well as a violinist, she subsequently recalled how her mother had given her *Violin: Six Lessons* one Christmas when she was fifteen or sixteen. She grew up in a relatively remote part of the country, and the book opened a new way of thinking about how to play the instrument. Through Menuhin's book, she learned the importance of establishing a "connection with your body as a first instrument," reflected on how none of her teachers had stressed this, and discovered that she found the "mind/body connection quite interesting."[14] Menuhin became one of her heroes as she studied and practiced his approach outlined in the book's instructions and diagrams. Senungetuk also credits Menuhin with introducing her to yoga through *Six Lessons*. While she does not claim to be a hard-core yoga practitioner today, she "returns to it as a constant,"[15] to bring her back to her body and to be centered, not just as a violinist but as a human being functioning in the world.

When she was an undergraduate music student, Senungetuk had the thrilling opportunity to meet Menuhin after a concert he conducted with the Warsaw Sinfonia in 1987. She recalls how Menuhin opened the concert with Bach's Violin Concerto No. 2 in E major BWV 1042 and performed as both the solo violinist and leader of the chamber orchestra. She found it to be a lovely and novel way to present the piece in his dual musical roles. To be able to hear him play the Bach—a piece she had studied—was doubly exciting. After the concert, with her copy of *Six Lessons* and a pen in hand, Senungetuk ran backstage to be first in line to meet Menuhin and to get his autograph. She recalls how his informal attire (his classic white sweater) made him more approachable and how he noticed that her book was worn and well-used. Years later, she found her concert program inside her copy of *Six Lessons*, and she still remembers how he was truly an inspiration to her.

In the end, Menuhin's yoga practice was about much more than fixing his violin technique, as he channeled the fruits of his practice to be an influence for good in our world. His life burned with passion and zeal when he performed, passed on his knowledge, and served humankind.

Eleanor Hope recalls Menuhin's relentless energy and how he couldn't bear to see blank pages in his calendar: "They had to be crammed full of something, and if it wasn't concerts, he was giving interviews or going off to see people or starting new projects. There was a restlessness, a drive in him, that was super-human . . . he was a gypsy: he could never stay in one place, was always on the move, looking to the next project, the next idea."[16]

As people from all walks of life, ranging from artists to business people and spiritual seekers to politicians, look for ways to balance the body/mind/spirit, may they look to the life and work of Yehudi Menuhin for a model. As a human being, he found yoga to be a means to improve his physical, emotional, and mental health. As a doer, he exerted refined and deliberate actions; as a thinker, he reflected on his experiences wisely; and as a spiritual seeker, he had faith in God, his guru, and his studies. In short, Menuhin's personality exhibited yoga *sattvic* qualities of equanimity such as nonviolence, truthfulness, and absence of anger; serenity and compassion for all beings; freedom from desire; and gentleness, modesty, and faithfulness.[17]

As his achievements and contributions to music and our world went well beyond correcting his violin technique through yoga, may we be inspired by the power of his practice to achieve such levels of competence, creativity, and health. And to those who also practice this now-popular discipline, may you also feel called to action, apply lessons learned on the yoga mat into your own daily life, and acquire the *sattvic* qualities that Menuhin exhibited. If we can harness such positive yoga energy, we can channel it as a powerful force for goodness as Menuhin did; we can effect positive changes in our world; and we can protect and heal our planet and people as we unleash a universal power of love and devotion.

Appendix

Archival Sources

Archival sources from the Foyle Menuhin Archive, Royal Academy of Music, London, visited in Mar. 2016, Mar. 2018, and Jan. 2020; the Ramamani Iyengar Memorial Yoga Institute (RIMYI) Archive, Pune, India, visited in Jan. 2018; and the Menuhin Center Saanen, Switzerland, visited in Jan. 2020.

Foyle Menuhin Archive

The extensive and comprehensive Foyle Menuhin Archive covers the life, career, and personal interests of Yehudi Menuhin. It was acquired by the Royal Academy of Music in March 2004, with generous funding from the Foyle Foundation and other donors. The archive consists of books, printed music, manuscripts, photographs, programs, correspondence, objets d'art, drawings, paintings, memorabilia, scrapbooks, and newspaper clippings. During my three visits to the archive, I worked through the boxes and folders marked "Yoga," "India and Indian Music," "Philosophy and Religion," and "Speeches and Addresses."

Letters in Chronological Order

Iyengar to Menuhin, Nov. 2, 1954.
Iyengar to Menuhin, n.d., but postmarked year looks like 1955.
Iyengar to Menuhin, June 1, 1955.
Iyengar to Menuhin, July 15, 1960.
Iyengar to Menuhin, July 23, 1960.
Menuhin to John G. Murray, July 28, 1960.

Menuhin to Iyengar, Nov. 8, 1961.

RIMYI letter to Menuhin July 5, 1978, requesting message for Iyengar's sixtieth birthday celebration in Dec. 1978.

Menuhin's sixtieth birthday message to Iyengar, 1978.

Menuhin to Dr. Satyanath, response to the BBC World Phone-In program, Nov. 4, 1983.

BBC to Menuhin, thank you letter for appearance in the World Phone-In, Nov. 7, 1983.

Festival of India organizer to Menuhin, requesting contribution to the publication planned in conjunction with the festival to be held in the US in 1985, Dec. 26, 1983.

Menuhin to Clifford Longley at *The Times*, Aug. 15, 1989.

Menuhin to Dr. Drury, dean of King's College, Feb. 1, 1991, in which he summarized his recent "Sermon on Music and Religion."

Menuhin to Ravi Shankar, n.d. (but the date was Oct. 14, 1994).

Iyengar to Menuhin, Nov. 7, 1995.

Iyengar to Menuhin, Dec. 23, 1995.

Iyengar to Menuhin Dec. 26, 1997.

Iyengar to Menuhin, Jan. 23, 1998.

Menuhin to Iyengar, Mar. 30, 1998.

Iyengar to Menuhin, Apr. 19, 1998, with photo demonstrating head stand with props.

Iyengar to Menuhin, June 3, 1998.

Iyengar to Menuhin, July 26, 1998.

Geeta Iyengar to Menuhin, Aug. 11, 1998.

H. Ralph Schumacher Jr., MD, professor of medicine at the School of Medicine, University of Pennsylvania, Iyengar's eightieth birthday message, Sept. 8, 1998.

George Rochberg, composer and Annenberg professor of the humanities, University of Pennsylvania, Iyengar's eightieth birthday message, Sept. 9, 1998.

Menuhin to Ravi Shankar, Jan. 1998.

Iyengar to Menuhin, Oct. 10, 1998.

Menuhin to Iyengar, Mar. 30, 1998.

Newspaper and Magazine Clippings in Chronological Order

"Menuhin in Delhi, Virtuoso Hails 'Yoga' Cult," *Times of India*, Feb. 21, 1952.

"The Twain Shall Meet," Menuhin's article for the *Saturday Review*, Jan. 31, 1953.

"Yehudi's Yoga, He Tries Twists to Help Him as Violinist," *Life Magazine*, Feb. 1953.

"Around the Town—Menuhin—The Artist and The Yogi" *Sunday Standard* (Bombay), Mar. 21, 1954.

"Clapping Out of Turn—Raj Bhavan Concert," *Times of India* (Bombay), Mar. 21, 1954, clipping from Moshe's scrapbook.

"Yoga Turns Yehudi Upside Down," *Arkansas Gazette*, Sept. 12, 1954.

"Yehudi Stands on His Head," *People Today*, Feb. 23, 1955.

"Yehudi is a Yogi," *Montreal Canada Star*, May 21, 1955.

"The Music of India, An Ancient Art Form," *New York Times*, Apr. 17, 1955.

"Visiting Musicians from India at the Museum of Modern Art," *New York Times*, n.d. [Apr. 1955].

"Indian and Western Music: An Attempt to Forecast Future Trends," *Hemisphere: An Asian-Australian Magazine*, Sydney, Australia, Apr. 1962.

"Mr. Ben Gurion Stands on Head," cartoon newspaper clipping, n.d. [*New York Times*, early 1960s?].

"From East to West," Menuhin's article in *Times Supplement on the Arts in the Commonwealth*, Sept. 13, 1965.

"Musical Living, Nine Words: Yehudi Menuhin's Definitions," sidebar of a magazine, *Music Insider*, n.d. [1971].

"Man: By Definition a Religious Animal: Of the Sacredness of Consciousness, Conscience and Choice," Menuhin's essay in *World Faiths Insight*, Spring 1981.

"Escape the Fate of the Dinosaur," *The Times*, Aug. 21, 1989, part 1 of Menuhin's essay "On Oneness."

"Pray for an Orphaned Race," *The Times*, Aug. 22, 1989, part 2 of Menuhin's essay "On Oneness."

"The Reification of Rhythm," Menuhin's review of *Indian Music and the West*, by Gerry Farrell, *Times Higher Education Supplement*, July 11, 1997.

Menuhin New Delhi concert ad for Jan. 26, 1998, *Times of India*, Jan. 20, 1998.

Photos in Chronological Order

Menuhin in *sirsasana* (Head Stand Pose), with Iyengar instructing, identified and dated by Diana Menuhin.

Menuhin and Iyengar, series of photos taken by Jacques Naegeli in Gstaad, 1954.

Iyengar with Zamira in *sirsasana*, Gstaad, 1954.

"Yehudi Menuhin and His Guru," BBC Interview with David Attenborough, Aug. 21, 1963.

Iyengar, Menuhin, and Upadhye (violin teacher), Prashant's recital, Bombay, 1969.

Menuhin and Iyengar, Bombay, 1969, practicing *pranayama* (breath control), shoulder stand, and backbend.

Menuhin performing head stand in Brussels at the Palace before or after a performance of *Messiah*, n.d. [1960s?].

Menuhin in head stand, Gstaad, 1979.

Menuhin in *padmasana* (Lotus Pose) in the *Heuschober* (haystack) behind his chalet, Gstaad, n.d. [mid-1980s].

Essays, Lectures, and Other Documents in Chronological Order

"Yehudi Menuhin, Marcelle Gazelle at the Piano, in Aid of the Prime Minister's National Relief Fund," poster advertising Menuhin's two violin recital dates in Delhi, India, on Feb. 28 and Mar. 4 and orchestral concert on Mar. 6, 1952.

Omnibus, typescript of the Ford Foundation program Mar. 16, 1955, Salt Lake City.

"The Music of India, an Ancient Art Form," manuscript, adapted from *New York Times* article, Apr. 17, 1955.

"Shanta Rao and the Dances of South India," Menuhin script, Museum of Modern Art, New York, Apr. 26, 1955.

"Art and Science as Related Concepts," lecture for the Royal Institution of Great Britain, Jan. 30, 1959; also translated into German in Apr. 1960.

"The Growing Interest of Western Nations in Indian Music and Dance," *Manchurian Guardian*, Oct. 28, 1959, revised for the Asia Society of New York and then reprinted in the journal *Indian Student*, 1960.

Menuhin interview with Aley Hasan on Indian Music, BBC, Nov. 17, 1960.

Memo regarding itinerary for visiting Indian musicians, n.d. [1960?].

"Improvisation," lecture given at London University, May 23, 1962.

"Yehudi Menuhin and His Guru," transcript of interview with David Attenborough, BBC, Aug. 21, 1963.

"Nehru," Menuhin tribute to the Prime Minister, n.d. [1964?].

Original manuscript of Menuhin's foreword to Iyengar's *Light on Yoga* (1964).

Yehudi Menuhin School student interview transcripts, 1964.

"The New Morality," Chutter Ede Lecture, National Union of Teachers, Mar. 30, 1965. Printed version in the *World Academy of Art and Science Newsletter*, Nov. 1966.

"An Attempt to Investigate Possible Influences of Indian Classical Music on Our Own Music in the Future," typescript dated 1966, but essentially the same as the essay printed in *Hemisphere: An Asian-Australian Magazine*, Sydney, Australia, Apr. 1962.

Musical manuscripts of Indian ragas in Menuhin's manuscript, Ravi Shankar's manuscript with an inscription to Menuhin, and a copyist's manuscript, n.d. [mid-1960s?].

"Mr. Menuhin's Notes for Sleeve of Record with Ravi Shankar," July 5, 1966.

East Meets West (Angel/EMI Stereo 36418), Menuhin's notes on the album recording.

"Education on the Menuhin Plan," article by Irving Kolodin, publication unknown, Nov. 27, 1965.

"Homage to Alaudin Khan," Menuhin's message in Ravi Shankar's program, Dec. 3, 1972.

"University of Madras Message in Celebration of the 81st Birthday of His Holiness Sri Chandrasekarendra Sarasvati," Menuhin's message, Nov. 1974.

"Man: By Definition a Religious Animal: Of the Sacredness of Consciousness, Conscience and Choice: The Francis Younghusband Memorial Lecture, World Congress of Faiths," typescript for Menuhin's lecture at the Jerusalem Chamber, Westminster Abbey, July 18, 1980. Printed version in *World Faiths Insight* (Spring 1981): 3–11.

Festival of India message, Menuhin's typescript message, n.d. [1985].

"Endless Time," unpublished paper, typescript, and manuscript. This appears to be a script for Menuhin's project on Indian art and culture, n.d.

"On Oneness," original manuscript, twenty typed pages, n.d. [1989]. Published in two installments in *The Times* (see clippings above) and also translated to German as "Eins-sein" by Helmut Viebrick, Sept. 1989 for Goethe Universität, Frankfurt, and to French by Mdme. Madeline Santschi, n.d.

"King's College: Music and Religion," Menuhin's handwritten notes for his "Sermon on Music and Religion," n.d. [Jan. 1991].

"My Prayer," four-page typescript, n.d., but enclosed with letter to Dr. Drury of Kings College, Feb. 1, 1991.

"The Meaning of Life," typescript, n.d. [1991?].

"The Meaning of Life," fax to *Life Magazine*, Aug. 20, 1991.
"The Meaning of Life," fax to Sichtermann International Publishing House, Oct. 16, 1991.
"Do You Believe in God?" Menuhin's answer to fifth-grade student Paul Rifkin from E. Sandwich, MA, n.d.
Menuhin eightieth birthday message to Iyengar [1998].

Documents on Human Rights in Chronological Order

Comments on trials in Russia in 1972 and 1973.
The imprisonment of Sakharcus (?) in 1984 and how Menuhin would cancel the concert planned for the tenth anniversary of Oistrak's death unless he was released.
Letter on the forced repatriation of the Vietnamese boat people, Nov. 29, 1980.
Letter to the editor of *The Times* on apartheid in South Africa and democratic process for blacks and whites, June 26, 1986.
Letter on genocide of the Kurds, 1991.
Speech on anti-Semitism made to UNESCO (in German), conference, June 13–24, 1992.

RAMAMANI IYENGAR MEMORIAL YOGA INSTITUTE

Description

The collection of the Menuhin documents is organized in a blue, two-holed notebook with a flexible wire binding. Each original document is followed by one to three photocopies. Most have small sticky notes with a JPEG file name of "Yehudi" and dates, which indicates these files have been scanned (I moved the sticky notes from the original documents to the copies in order to protect the originals). Most documents are numbered in reverse chronological order, but the documents in the binder are in (more or less) chronological order from the beginning (* indicates out of chronological order).

Contents in Order of Binder

Summary of eight letters (unsigned) on three hand-written unbound pages, dated Aug. 7, 2016 (probably compiled to prepare for the

Yoga Rahasya Menuhin Centenary Issue 23/2, 2016); May 20, 1954; Dec. 8, 1954; Nov. 27, 1956; Sept. 25, 1957; Sept. 16, 1965; Feb. 23, 1966; Sept. 30, 1974; and Aug. 22, 1995.

[Unnumbered]* Message from Lord Menuhin to B. K. S. Iyengar (B. K. S. I.) on his eightieth birthday celebration (1998) in plastic cover, unbound.

32.* Honorary Knighthood card (from 1965); thank you to B. K. S. Iyengar for sending his congratulations.

31. Menuhin to Iyengar, 1952, Mar. 7—Government Bombay House [Menuhin's first trip to India].

30.* Menuhin to Iyengar, 1952, Mar. 5—Government Bombay House.

29. Menuhin to Iyengar, 1954, May 20—from 41 West Hill Highgate 6 [after Menuhin's second trip to India]; impact of yoga on his violin playing; first invitation to B. K. S. I. to come to Gstaad.

28. Menuhin to Iyengar, 1954, Dec. 8—from 41 West Hill Highgate 6; note of thanks; results of yoga work.

27. Menuhin to Iyengar, 1955, Nov. 23—on onion skin paper, from Claridge Hotel, Brook St., London; regarding Gstaad.

26. Menuhin to Iyengar, 1956, Nov. 27—on onion skin paper, from Cape Town, South Africa; following Y. M.'s back surgery.

25. Menuhin to Iyengar, 1957, Sept. 25—on onion skin paper, from Chalet Wasserngrat, Gstaad; to Mr. Paton, with following message of introduction of B. K. S. I.; had forwarded to B. K. S. I. with added note at bottom of letter.

24. Menuhin to Iyengar, 1960, Jan. 4—on blue stationery, c/o Harold Holt, Ltd., typed; plans to bring B. K. S. I. to London.

23. Menuhin to Iyengar, 1961, Jan. 7—on blue stationery with engraved address 2. The Grove, Highgate Village, London, No. 6; handwritten.

22. Menuhin to Iyengar, 1961, Dec. 29—on Highgate Village stationery.

21. Menuhin to Iyengar, 1961, April 18—on Highgate Village stationery.

20. Menuhin to Iyengar, 1962, Jan. 28, on Raj Bhavan stationery, handwritten; recommendation for B. K. S. I.'s passport renewal [Menuhin's third trip to India].

19. Menuhin to Iyengar, 1962, Feb. 9—on Raj Bhavan stationery, handwritten; thank you to Mrs. Iyengar.

18. Menuhin to Iyengar, 1962, Mar. 21—on Hotel Windsor stationery (Melbourne), handwritten; follow-up on recent work together in India.

17. Menuhin to Iyengar, 1962, Dec. 23—on Highgate stationery, typed; response to B. K. S. I.'s dream.

16. Menuhin to Iyengar, 1963, April 19—on Highgate stationery, typed; opening of Menuhin's school; mentions Prashant's violin; another invitation to Gstaad.

15. Menuhin to Iyengar, 1965, Sept. 16—on Highgate stationery, typed; after return from Greece, references to Queen and Prashant playing violin; Prashant's second violin; playing with Indian musicians at Commonwealth Arts Festival; yoga progress; sympathy for political problems in India.

14.* [?] to Iyengar, 1965, Sept. 3—picture postcard from Altersee [I am quite positive this postcard is from Clifford Curzon, not Menuhin].

13. Menuhin to Iyengar, 1966, Feb. 23—on Privatklinik, Zurich, stationery, handwritten; *Light on Yoga* is "gift to the whole world"; practicing "exercises" daily.

12. Menuhin to Iyengar, 1966, Dec. 28—on plain stationery, handwritten; update letter on news.

11. Menuhin to Iyengar, 1967, Nov. 29—on the Drake Hotel, NY, stationery; will contribute words to French film on B. K. S. I.'s work; asks if coming to Gstaad again next summer.

10. Menuhin to Iyengar, 1968, April 11—on blue Highgate stationery, typed, with attached letter to Prime Minister Indira Gandhi outlining his BBC India project vision.

9. Menuhin to Iyengar, 1969, Aug. 20—plain notepad paper, handwritten [Gstaad?]; reference to B. K. S. I. working with the boys; will keep up his work, especially the right shoulder.

8. Menuhin to Iyengar, 1972, June 2—onion skin paper, typed; to London Centre of Bharatiya Vidya Bhavan.

7. Menuhin to Mr. Lobo, 1974, Sept. 30—blue Highgate stationery, typed; regarding inauguration of RIMYI.

6. Menuhin's text for the RIMYI inauguration, 1974, Nov. 22.

5. Menuhin to Iyengar, 1980, Oct. 30—white Highgate stationery, handwritten; response to B. K. S. I. letter from Oct. 20; reports and reflections.

4. Menuhin to Iyengar, 1995, Oct. 28—on the Taj Mahal, Bombay, stationery; shaky handwriting, memories of Government House forty years back; greetings but cannot come to visit.

[4a.]* Menuhin to Dr. Mehta, 1995, Aug. 22—stapled together with no. 4., on Chalet Chankly Bone, Gstaad, stationery; regarding receipt of the [first?] *Yoga Rahasya* issue.

3. Menuhin to Iyengar, 1995, Dec. 8—on Lord Menuhin, 65 Chester Square, London, stationery, typed; regarding B. K. S. I.'s hurt feelings for Y. M. not visiting while in Bombay.

2. Menuhin to Iyengar, 1998, May 20—on Lord Menuhin stationery, typed; thank you for B. K. S. I.'s advice and photos of *asanas* to practice; beginning to do his "exercises" again; relationship repaired.

1. Menuhin to Iyengar, 1998, Sept. 21 (numbered 33 in upper righthand corner of the original, but 1 on photo copy)—thanks for sending photos of *asanas* to practice; apologies for not being able to attend eightieth birthday celebration.

MENUHIN CENTER SAANEN

"Ausstellung im Festival-Zelt: The Maestro's Master Yehudi Menuhin's Best Violin Teacher, B. K. S. Iyengar," program reprinted photos from Aug. 11, 1962, and the program of activities on Sept. 3 and 4, 2004.

Yoga Vidya, Bulletin 2004, commemorative booklet of articles and programs from Iyengar's visits to Switzerland for the celebration of fifty years of yoga in Switzerland, Gstaad, 2004, Iyengar-Yoga-Vereinigung Schweiz, Iyengar Yoga, Switzerland.

Various Large Posters of Menuhin and Iyengar in Gstaad

Commemorative frame of concert poster for Menuhin's debut concert with Bruno Walter in Berlin, Apr. 12, 1929.

Notes

Notes to the Introduction

1. Bruno Monsaingeon, *Passion Menuhin: The Album of a Life*. Berlin: EuroArts Music International, 2016. Published with *The Menuhin Century*. Warner Classics 0825646777068, 2016. The extensive collection includes eighty CDs and eleven DVDs; see https://www.warnerclassics.com/artist/menuhin-century.

2. I'm grateful to my brother Don Wendland, who also practices yoga, for planting the seed in my mind for this important point during a conversation in June 2019 while on a trip in the Red River Gorge, Kentucky.

Notes to Chapter 1

1. Today the city is called Mumbai, but I will refer to it by its former name, as Iyengar and Menuhin do.

2. B. K. S. Iyengar, "The Historic Meeting," *Yoga Rahasya* 23/2 (2016): 9–10.

3. Yehudi Menuhin, *Unfinished Journey: Twenty Years Later* (New York: Fromm International Publishing, 1997), 259.

4. Menuhin, 259.

5. Menuhin, 259.

6. "Events and News," *United Nations* (website), accessed June 7, 2019, https://www.un.org/en/events/yogaday/background.shtml.

7. Yoga Journal editors, "New Study Finds More Than 20 Million Yogis in U.S.," *Yoga Journal*, Dec. 5, 2012, https://www.yogajournal.com/blog/new-study-finds-20-million-yogis-u-s.

8. Taffy Brodesser-Akner, "How Kelli O'Hara Gets Ready for Broadway, Night After Night," *New York Times Magazine*, June 2, 2019, 16.

9. "23 Celebrities Who Swear By Yoga," *YogiApproved* (website), accessed Sept. 23, 2019, https://www.yogiapproved.com/yoga/22-celebrities-yoga-fanatics/.

10. The other five schools of thought include Samkhya, Nyaya, Vaishesika,

Mimamsa, and Vedanta.

11. For a detailed discussion of the meaning and interpretation of the word "yoga," see David Gordon White, *The Yoga Sutra of Patañjali: A Biography* (Princeton, NJ: Princeton University Press, 2014), 1–15.

12. For further reading, see the bibliography for references to some of these sources, including those by Chappell, Goldberg, De Michelis, Newcombe, Sarbacker, and Singleton. I found Sarbacker's most recent book, *Tracing the Path of Yoga* (Albany: State University of New York Press, 2021), to be especially helpful, as the author's tone targets both yoga scholars and the educated layperson. See especially chapter 1, "Defining Yoga," 9–38, where he maps out common threads within the various strands in Indian religion and philosophy rather than trying to define yoga in essentialist terms.

13. Elizabeth De Michelis, *A History of Modern Yoga: Patañjali and Western Esotericism* (New York: Continuum, 2005), 2–3.

14. De Michelis, 2.

15. Suzanne Newcombe, *Yoga in Britain: Stretching Spirituality and Educating Yogis* (Sheffield, UK: Equinox Publishing, 2019), 24.

16. David Gordon White, *The Yoga Sutra of Patañjali*, 192–94. White cites a passage from Yeats's introduction to a 1937 translation of Patañjali's work and references a passage from Eliot's *The Waste Land* that can be interpreted through the lens of "Patañajali's analysis of subliminal impressions and the seeds of karma from past lives."

17. Newcombe, *Yoga in Britain*, 118–19.

18. For example, see the discussion in De Michelis, *A History of Modern Yoga*, 194 ff.

19. Newcombe, *Yoga in Britain*, 94. Interestingly, Menuhin's sister, Hephzibah Hauser, played a crucial role in bringing Iyengar to this position. She mentioned how much she benefited from the guru's instruction to the head of the physical education in ILEA, Peter McIntosh, at a social event, which in turn led McIntosh to investigate Iyengar and his work. See Newcombe, *Yoga in Britain*, 96.

20. For further reading on how Western, especially European, Orientalists in the late nineteenth and first decades of the twentieth centuries shaped this status of Patañjali and the *Yoga Sutras*, see Mark Singleton, "The Classical Reveries of Modern Yoga: Patanjali and Constructive Orientalism," in *Yoga in the Modern World: A Contemporary Perspective* (London: Routledge, 2008), 77–99.

21. Gudrun Bühnemann, "Naga, Siddha and Sage: Visions of Patañjali as an Authority on Yoga," in *Yoga in Transformation*, eds. Karl Baier, Philipp A. Maas, and Karin Preisendanz (Vienna: Vienna University Press, 2018), 578.

22. Singleton, "The Classical Reveries of Modern Yoga," 91.

23. B. K. S. Iyengar, *Light on the Yoga Sutras* (London: Thorsons, 1996), 49–50. Unless otherwise noted, I am using Iyengar's translations of yoga terms throughout this book.

24. Edwin F. Bryant, *The Yoga Sutras of Patañjali* (New York: North Point

Press, 2009), 169.

25. Both *kriyayoga* from Patanjali's *Yoga Sutras* and *karmayoga* from the *Bhagavad Gita* are translated as Yoga of Action.

26. B. K. S. Iyengar, *Astadala Yogamala, Vol. 1* (New Delhi, India: Allied Publisher, 2000), 20.

27. De Michelis, *A History of Modern Yoga*, 195.

28. Iyengar, *Astadala Yogamala*, 15–16.

29. The Samkhya tradition is broadly theistic, allowing for many names of *isvara* (God), and dualistic, in that it recognizes two independent realities, *purusa* (pure consciousness) and *prakriti* (matter). It holds that ignorance results from mistaking *prakriti* for *purusa*, which in turn creates suffering, and liberation from this bondage reveals the true self. While *purusa* stands alone as the true self/soul, *prakriti* is everything else in the universe. It is laid out in twenty-four constituents from primordial matter to three components of consciousness (intelligence, ego, and mind); five organs of perception (ears, skin, eyes, tongue, and nose); five organs of action (mouth, arms, legs, excretory, and reproductive); five sense elements (sound, touch, sight, taste, and smell); and five gross elements (ether/space, air, fire, water, and earth). It postulates three *gunas* (forces or tendencies) that influence all of *prakrti*, namely *tamas* (inertia), *rajas* (dynamism, vitality), and *sattva* (equanimity, luminosity) and recognizes three means to acquire knowledge, namely perception, inference, and reliable sources. See "Table 9: *The Evolution and Involution of* Prakrti" in *Light on the Yoga Sutras*, by B. K. S. Iyengar, 132–33; and "Samkhya Evolution of Prakrti," *Yoga St. Louis Blog*, accessed July 14, 2020, https://yogastlouisblog.files.wordpress.com/2013/09/samkhya-cosmogenychartcolor-lowresconv.jpg.

30. Kausthub Desikachar, prologue to *Yoga Makiranda*, by Tirumalai Krishnamacharya, trans. and ed. T. V. K. Desikachar (Chennai, India: MediaGaruda, 2011), 17. When describing his own yoga lineage, Iyengar also references Krishnamacharya's studies with Brahmachari in *Astadala Yogamala*, 28.

31. A. G. Mohan, *Krishnamacharya: His Life and Teachings* (Boston: Shambala Publications, 2010), 29.

32. Krishnamacharya, *Yoga Makiranda*, 68, n. 24.

33. Other yoga masters close to Iyengar's age who trained with Krishnamacharya include Indra Devi (1899–2002), who became "the first lady of yoga" in the US after World War II, and K. Pattabhi Jois (1915–2009), who subsequently established Ashtanga Yoga. Later notable students include Krishnamacharya's son T. K. V. Desikachar (b. 1938) and Srivatsa Ramaswami (b. 1939).

34. Iyengar, *Astadala Yogamala*, 28–29.

35. Much later in life, Iyengar detailed how he struggled to master *pranayama* for over twenty years and how his guru refused to teach him the practice when he was a student. Iyengar, "How I Learnt *Pranayama*," in *Astadala Yogamala*, 64. In 1985, Iyengar even credited Menuhin for being an

indirect guru from whom I learnt the placing of the fingers very accurately on the nostril passages, though he never knew that I learned from him. I observed his fingering work, the mobility of the knuckles on the violin strings and the placement of the tip of the thumb on the bow and fingers on the strings. This gave me the clue of placing the thumb and fingers on the nose to control the inner carpet of the membranes and to trace the exact air passage for my *pranayama*. (Iyengar, *Astadala Yogamala*, 64)

36. B. K. S. Iyengar, *Light on Life: The Yoga Journey to Wholeness, Inner Peace, and Ultimate Freedom* ([Emmaus, PA]: Rodale Books, 2005), 71–72.

37. Jake Clennell, dir., *Iyengar: The Man, Yoga, and the Student's Journey* (Clennell Films, 2018). Documentary film. For details, see http://iyengarmovie.com/.

38. For example, see "B. K. S Iyengar 1938 Newsreel Part 1 (Silent)," YouTube, https://www.youtube.com/watch?v=lmOUZQi_6Tw&t=40s, or search "Iyengar 1938 video."

39. Clennell, *Iyengar: The Man, Yoga, and the Student's Journey.*

40. De Michelis, *A History of Modern Yoga*, 197.

41. De Michelis, 198, as quoted in Anne Cushman, "Iyengar Looks Back," *Yoga Journal* 137 (1997): 158.

42. De Michelis, 198.

43. For example, Iyengar said in a 1984 lecture/demonstration at Davies Symphony Hall in San Francisco: "As an artist on the platform, as a performer, I have to curtail words and present my practice through direct perception, so that you can receive how the self can radiate through its vehicle, the body." Iyengar, "Self Analysis and Yoga," in *Astadala Yogamala*, 79.

44. Iyengar, 203–4.

45. Rolf Steiger, director of the Menuhin Center in Saanen, interview by the author, Jan. 3, 2020, as we walked together on the "philosopher's path" between Saanen and Gstaad.

46. Kofi Busia, "B. K. S. Iyengar Biography," *Kofi Busia* (website), accessed July 3, 2018, http://www.kofibusia.com/iyengarbiography/iyengarbio14.php.

47. De Michelis, *A History of Modern Yoga*, 203.

48. B. K. S. Iyengar, *Light on Yoga*, rev. ed. (New York: Schocken Books, 1979), 19. The author cited by Iyengar here is Mahadev Desai in his introduction to the *Gita according to Gandhi*.

49. Iyengar, 19.

50. Iyengar, 22. Iyengar compares yoga to music in other metaphorical statements, most famously, "Yoga is like music: the rhythm of the body, the melody of the mind, and the harmony of the soul create the symphony of life."

51. Iyengar, 20.

52. Iyengar, 28.

53. Later in his life, Iyengar maintained this was the yoga he taught: "The Yoga I teach is purely *astangayoga*, known as the eight limbs of yoga, expounded by Patanjali in the 196 sutras each of which reflects profound experimental knowledge supplemented with Hatha Yoga texts, Gita and others." "Guruji on Iyengar Yoga," *Yoga Rahasya* 27/1 (2020): 23.

54. "Guruji on Iyengar Yoga," 41.

55. Guruji B. K. S. Iyengar, "Light on *Light on Yoga*," *Yoga Rahasya* 23/3 (2016): 9.

56. For an online PDF of the 1980 condensed edition, see "Iyengar BKS: The Illustrated *Light on Yoga*," *Academia* (website), accessed Sept. 3, 2022, https://www.academia.edu/25481532/Iyengar_B_K_S_The_Illustrated_Light_On_Yoga.

57. De Michelis, *A History of Modern Yoga*, 201.

58. Thanks to yoga scholar Suzanne Newcombe for this idea, in conversation at the Flask, a landmark restaurant near Menuhin's former residence in Highgate, London, Jan. 7, 2020.

59. For further discussion of how *kriyayoga* provides a "capsule" for these three paths, including references to the *Bhagavad Gita*, see Iyengar, *Light on the Yoga Sutras*, 6–7, 109, and the chart on 110; and Bryant, *The Yoga Sutras of Patañjali*, 171–73.

60. Robin Daniels, *Conversations with Menuhin* (New York: St. Martin's Press, 1979), 185.

61. Daniels, 69.

62. Iyengar, *Light on Life*, 87.

63. Iyengar writes how he wanted to be an artist in his yoga practice and was inspired as a young man after "first seeing the beautiful hands of Yehudi Menuhin." Iyengar, *Light on Life*, 264–65.

64. Iyengar, 265.

65. Menuhin, *Unfinished Journey*, 258.

66. Menuhin, 257.

67. Menuhin, 257.

68. Menuhin, 258.

69. Menuhin, 258.

70. Menuhin, 259.

71. "Interview with Sri Prashant Iyengar on Yehudi Menuhin," *Yoga Rahasya* 23/2, Menuhin Centenary Issue (2016): 35.

72. Iyengar, *Light on the Yoga Sutras*, xvii.

73. Yehudi Menuhin, "The Words," *Yehudi Menuhin* (website), accessed July 15, 2021, https://www.menuhin.org/the-words.

74. As of this writing, seventy-nine countries have a total of 5,824 certified Iyengar teachers, with the majority by far in the UK and the US. "Number of Certified Iyengar Yoga Teachers," *bksiyengar.com*, accessed July 3, 2019, http://bksiyengar.com/modules/Iyoga/noteach.htm.

75. Menuhin letter to Iyengar, Mar. 5, 1952, Ramamani Iyengar Memorial Yoga Institute (RIMYI) Archive, Pune, India.

76. Menuhin letter to Iyengar, Mar. 7, 1952, RIMYI Archive.

77. Rujuta Diwekar, "'You Have Taught Me How to Play the Violin,'" interview with B. K. S. Iyengar, *Bangalore Mirror*, updated Aug. 20, 2014, https://bangaloremirror.indiatimes.com/news/india/Yehudi-Menuhin-greatest-violinistsB-K-S-Iyengar/articleshow/40525332.cms.

78. Harsh Desai, "Light on the Life of a Master," interview with B. K. S. Iyengar, *Spectrum: The Tribune*, Dec. 4, 2005, http://www.tribuneindia.com/2005/20051204/spectrum/main1.htm.

79. Iyengar says this in both interviews cited above.

80. Menuhin, *Unfinished Journey*, 259.

81. *Organizer Delhi* clipping, Apr. 5, 1954, Foyle Menuhin Archive, Royal Academy of Music, London.

82. *Organizer Delhi*.

83. Desai, "Light on the Life of a Master."

84. Menuhin letter to Iyengar, May 20, 1954, RIMYI Archive.

85. Menuhin letter to Iyengar.

86. According to Rolf Steiger, Menuhin stayed at this hotel. Steiger interview with the author, Gstaad, Jan. 3, 2020.

87. Iyengar, *Astadala Yogamala*, 47.

88. Iyengar, "The Historic Meeting," 12.

89. Iyengar letter to Menuhin, Nov. 2, 1954, Foyle Menuhin Archive.

90. Menuhin letter to Iyengar, Dec. 8, 1954, RIMYI Archive.

91. Iyengar letter to Menuhin, n.d., but postmarked year looks like 1955, Foyle Menuhin Archive.

92. Iyengar letter to Menuhin, June 1, 1955, Foyle Menuhin Archive.

93. Zamira began to live with Yehudi and Diana Menuhin when she was thirteen, but his son Krov stayed with mother Nola throughout his teenage years. Humphrey Burton, *Menuhin: A Life* (London: Faber and Faber, 2000), 338.

94. Menuhin letter to Iyengar, Nov. 23, 1955, RIMYI Archive.

95. Elliott Goldberg, *The Path of Modern Yoga: The History of an Embodied Spiritual Practice* (Rochester, VT: Inner Traditions, 2016), 381.

96. This was Menuhin's third visit to South Africa, where he participated in the Johannesburg Festival, but he was not to go again until the end of apartheid.

97. Menuhin letter to Iyengar, Nov. 27, 1956, RIMYI Archive.

98. Menuhin letter to Iyengar, Nov. 8, 1961, Foyle Menuhin Archive. Although the correspondence provides no further details about the sufferers of Bihar, it most like refers to the caste rivalries and political struggles in that northern Indian state.

99. Menuhin letter to Iyengar.

100. Letter from Menuhin "To Whom it May Concern" in support of Iyengar's application for passport renewal, Jan. 28, 1962, RIMYI Archive.

101. Menuhin letter to Mrs. Iyengar, Feb. 9, 1962, RIMYI Archive.

102. "Interview with Sri Prashant Iyengar on Yehudi Menuhin," *Yoga Rahasya* 23/2 (2016): 33.

103. "Interview with Sri Prashant Iyengar," 33.

104. "Interview with Sri Prashant Iyengar," 34. Note Prashant cites the year as 1964 in this article, but Menuhin mentions the new violin in his Sept. 16, 1965, letter to Iyengar.

105. "Interview with Sri Prashant Iyengar," 34.

106. Menuhin letter to Iyengar, Apr. 19, 1963, RIMYI Archive.

107. Menuhin letter to Iyengar, Mar. 21, 1962, RIMYI Archive.

108. Menuhin letter to Iyengar, Mar. 21.

109. Menuhin letter to Iyengar, Mar. 21.

110. Menuhin letter to Iyengar, Dec. 23, 1962, RIMYI Archive.

111. Menuhin letter to Iyengar, Dec. 23.

112. The manuscript was typed by two devotees of Menuhin who were active in his London-based Asian Music Circle, Angela Marris and Beatrice Harthan, who brought the manuscript to the attention of an editor at Allen & Unwin publishers Gerald Yorke, who was interested in sourcing Indian and esoteric books. See Newcombe, *Yoga in Britain*, 28–29, 92–93.

113. Menuhin letter to John G. Murray, July 28, 1960, Foyle Menuhin Archive.

114. Menuhin, *Unfinished Journey*, 261.

115. All the following quotes come from Yehudi Menuhin, foreword to *Light on Yoga*, B. K. S. Iyengar, 11–12.

116. Many thanks to Suzanne Newcombe for sending me the interview transcript from when she talked with Angela Marris before she died and a letter she sent with the Beatrice Harthan speech at a 1993 Euroyoga convention to introduce Iyengar. Angela Marris made it clear to Newcombe that her primary interest was being close to Menuhin not Iyengar, whereas Beatrice Harthan was more interested in helping Iyengar. Additionally, Newcombe reported there were many letters in the Reading Archives between Harthan and Yorke about Iyengar in the 1970s, as Harthan continued to arrange Iyengar's accommodations throughout that decade.

117. Newcombe, *Yoga in Britain*, 34.

118. Rolf Steiger and Hans-Ulrich Tschanz, *Gstaad und die Menuhins* (Wabern-Bern: Benteli Verlags AG, 2006), 32.

119. Menuhin letter to Iyengar, Sept. 16, 1965, RIMYI Archive. This was a prophetic suggestion, since Iyengar's children Geeta and Prashant would later take over as codirectors of RIMYI and advance their father's legacy.

120. Menuhin's sixtieth birthday message to Iyengar, 1978, Foyle Menuhin Archive.

121. Menuhin's sixtieth birthday message to Iyengar.

122. Menuhin letter to Iyengar, Oct. 30, 1980, RIMYI Archive.

123. Menuhin greeting to Iyengar for his seventieth birthday, 1988, Foyle Menuhin Archive.

124. Menuhin letter to Iyengar, Oct. 29, 1995, RIMYI Archive.

125. Although Menuhin wrote Iyengar while in Bombay to convey his greetings, Iyengar's feelings were hurt because Menuhin did not make the effort to see him. Iyengar also had doubts Menuhin had actually been reading his previous letters, since at times his secretary had responded. Menuhin assured Iyengar that he had read them all but owing to his busy schedule had not always been able to reply personally. As for not seeing each other in October in India, Menuhin asked his dear friend to "not entertain feelings of offence or hurt. Diana's and my days in India were so full and it was our own private holiday that it was absolutely impossible for me to find any time for our wonderful work, which I remember from 40 years back." Menuhin letter to Iyengar, Dec. 8, 1995, RIMYI Archive. Iyengar closed this misunderstanding a couple of weeks later, saying he too regretted that Menuhin felt hurt by his letter, and he hastened to assure Menuhin his affections had not faded at all. Fittingly, Iyengar let go of any ill-feelings and wrote, "If God wills who knows we may meet somewhere on the Planet again." Iyengar letter to Menuhin, Dec. 23, 1995, Foyle Menuhin Archive.

126. Manouso Manos, conversation with the author in Atlanta, GA, Aug. 2, 2016.

127. Iyengar letter to Menuhin, Jan. 23, 1998, Foyle Menuhin Archive.

128. Iyengar letter to Menuhin, Jan. 23.

129. Iyengar letter to Menuhin, Apr. 19, 1998, Foyle Menuhin Archive.

130. Menuhin letter to Iyengar, May 20, 1998, RIMYI Archive.

131. Iyengar letter to Menuhin June 3, 1998, Foyle Menuhin Archive.

132. Iyengar letter to Menuhin, July 26, 1998, Foyle Menuhin Archive.

133. Geeta Iyengar letter to Menuhin, Aug. 11, 1998, Foyle Menuhin Archive.

134. Menuhin letter to Iyengar, Sept. 21, 1998, RIMYI Archive.

135. Menuhin letter to Iyengar, Sept. 21.

136. Menuhin's eightieth birthday message to Iyengar, RIMYI and Foyle Menuhin Archives.

137. Iyengar letter to Menuhin, Oct. 10, 1998, Foyle Menuhin Archive.

138. Menuhin, *Unfinished Journey*, 263.

139. Menuhin, 263.

Notes to Chapter 2

1. Yehudi Menuhin, *Unfinished Journey: Twenty Years Later* (New York: Fromm International Publishing, 1997), 9.

2. Menuhin, 67.

3. Robert Magidoff, *Yehudi Menuhin*, 2nd ed. (London: Robert Hale, 1973), 135–36.

4. Magidoff, 124.

5. Magidoff, 136.

6. Magidoff, 171.

7. Menuhin, *Unfinished Journey*, 134.

8. Menuhin, 66.

9. Robin Daniels, *Conversations with Menuhin* (New York: St. Martin's Press, 1979), 182.

10. Menuhin, *Unfinished Journey*, 57.

11. Menuhin, 68–69.

12. Menuhin, 72.

13. Menuhin, 80.

14. Menuhin, 82.

15. Yehudi Menuhin, *Life Class: Thoughts, Exercises, Reflections of an Itinerant Violinist* (London: Heinemann, 1986), 13.

16. This is how Menuhin referred to the folk music of Romania that Enesco introduced him to throughout his writings. While I believe Menuhin would be sensitive to how the descriptor is considered offensive to the Roma people today and would use the recommended Romani/Romany instead (https://www.merri-am-webster.com/dictionary/Gypsy#usage), he used the term in a positive way.

17. Magidoff, *Yehudi Menuhin*, 68.

18. Menuhin, *Unfinished Journey*, 134.

19. Menuhin, 131.

20. Magidoff, *Yehudi Menuhin*, 139.

21. Menuhin, *Unfinished Journey*, 120.

22. Magidoff, *Yehudi Menuhin*, 165.

23. Magidoff, 168.

24. Menuhin, *Unfinished Journey*, 147.

25. Menuhin, 148.

26. Magidoff, *Yehudi Menuhin*, 179.

27. Magidoff, 179.

28. Magidoff, 180.

29. Magidoff, 180.

30. Magidoff, 181.

31. Magidoff, 180.

32. Humphrey Burton, *Menuhin: A Life* (London: Faber and Faber, 2000), 184.

33. Menuhin, *Unfinished Journey*, 150.

34. Menuhin, 155.

35. Menuhin, 158.

36. Menuhin, 161.

37. Magidoff, *Yehudi Menuhin*, 206–7.

38. Menuhin, *Unfinished Journey*, 161.

39. Menuhin, 158.

40. Menuhin, 158.

41. Menuhin, 158.
42. Magidoff, *Yehudi Menuhin*, 203.
43. Menuhin, *Unfinished Journey*, 158.
44. Menuhin, 167.
45. Menuhin, 167.
46. Magidoff, *Yehudi Menuhin*, 222.
47. Menuhin, *Unfinished Journey*, 167.
48. Menuhin, 168.
49. Menuhin, 168–69.
50. Menuhin, 165.
51. Menuhin, 158.
52. Menuhin, 166–67.
53. Menuhin, 198.
54. Menuhin, 186.
55. Diana Menuhin, *Fiddler's Moll* (New York: St. Martin's Press, 1984), 30.
56. Magidoff, *Yehudi Menuhin*, 225.
57. Menuhin, *Unfinished Journey*, 198.
58. Menuhin, 185.
59. Menuhin, 190.
60. Menuhin, 190.
61. Menuhin, 223.
62. Menuhin, 223.
63. Menuhin, 227.
64. Menuhin, 229.
65. Menuhin, 234.
66. Menuhin, quoted in Magidoff, *Yehuhi Menuhin*, 250.
67. Menuhin, *Unfinished Journey*, 233.
68. Menuhin, 234–35.
69. Magidoff, *Yehuhi Menuhin*, 247.
70. Menuhin, *Unfinished Journey*, 235.
71. Menuhin, 236.
72. Menuhin, 236.
73. Menuhin, 236.
74. Menuhin, 236.
75. Menuhin, 237.
76. Menuhin, 238.
77. Menuhin, 239.
78. Menuhin, 247.
79. Menuhin, 254.
80. Menuhin, 262.
81. Menuhin, 260.

82. Yehudi Menuhin and William Primrose, *Yehudi Menuhin Music Guides: The Violin and Viola* (New York: Schirmer Books, 1976), 21.

Notes to Chapter 3

1. While *dharma* is a complex concept in Hindu philosophy, it can generally be understood to mean duty, responsibility, and purpose in one's life according to spiritual values.

2. Robin Daniels, *Conversations with Menuhin* (New York: St. Martin's Press, 1979), 80.

3. Daniels, 60.

4. Howard Taubman quoted in Humphrey Burton, *Menuhin: A Life* (London: Faber and Faber, 2000), 336.

5. "Yehudi's Yoga: He Tries Twists to Help Him as Violinist," *Life Magazine*, February 1953, Foyle Menuhin Archive, Royal Academy of Music, London.

6. *The Sunday Standard* (Bombay), Mar. 21, 1954, Foyle Menuhin Archive.

7. Respectively in the *Arkansas Gazette* (Sept. 12, 1954), *People Today* (Feb. 23, 1955), and the *Montreal Canada Star* (May 21, 1955), Foyle Menuhin Archive.

8. "Yehudi is a Yogi," *Montreal Canada Star*, May 21, 1955, Foyle Menuhin Archive.

9. Yehudi Menuhin, *Unfinished Journey: Twenty Years Later* (New York: Fromm International Publishing), 301. Note: the first was Indian Prime Minister Nehru in 1952.

10. Undated cartoon newspaper clipping, Foyle Menuhin Archive.

11. Menuhin, *Unfinished Journey*, 363.

12. Menuhin, 358.

13. Menuhin, 358.

14. Suzanne Newcombe, *Yoga in Britain: Stretching Spirituality and Educating Yogis* (Sheffield, UK: Equinox Publishing, 2019), 92–93.

15. Burton, *Menuhin*, 489–90.

16. See the festival website, https://www.gstaadmenuhinfestival.ch/en.

17. Diana Menuhin, *Fiddler's Moll* (New York: St. Martin's Press, 1984), 101.

18. Menuhin, 101.

19. Menuhin, *Unfinished Journey*, 359.

20. Menuhin, 360.

21. Menuhin letter to Iyengar, Sept. 16, 1965, RIMYI Archive, Pune, India.

22. Menuhin, *Unfinished Journey*, 270.

23. B. K. S. Iyengar, "The Historic Meeting," *Yoga Rahasya* 23/2 (2016): 11.

24. Iyengar, 29, 40, 45.

25. For this fascinating history, see Newcombe, *Yoga in Britain*, 40–74.

26. "Remembering Mr. Iyengar," *Yoga Rahasya* 23/2 (2016): 38.

27. Kofi Busia, "B. K. S. Iyengar Biography," *Kofi Busia* (website), accessed July 3, 2018, http://www.kofibusia.com/iyengarbiography/iyengarbio14.php.

28. See Iyengar's own explanation about his teaching approach and clips from a later demonstration in "CNN Interview with B. K. S. Iyengar," interview with Anjali Rao, *CNN Talk Asia*, June 3, 2012, YouTube video, 5:28–6:55, https://www.youtube.com/watch?v=cXJEzPGZqo8.

29. Newcombe, *Yoga in Britain*, 76.

30. Newcombe, 86.

31. Iyengar, "CNN Interview with B. K. S. Iyengar," 2:40–3:40, https://www.youtube.com/watch?v=cXJEzPGZqo8.

32. Iyengar, 2:40–3:40.

33. Suzanne Newcombe, "Spaces of Yoga: Towards a Non-Essentialist Understanding of Yoga," in *Yoga in Transformation: Historical and Contemporary Perspectives*, eds. Karl Baier, Philip A. Maas, and Karen Preisendanz (Göttingen: V&R unipress, Vienna University Press, 2018), 554, https://www.vandenhoeck-ruprecht-verlage.com/themen-entdecken/theologie/religionswissenschaft/16133/yoga-in-transformation.

34. B. K. S. Iyengar, *Light on Life: The Yoga Journey to Wholeness, Inner Peace, and Ultimate Freedom* ([Emmaus, PA]: Rodale Books, 2005), 175.

35. Elizabeth De Michelis, *A History of Modern: Yoga Patañjali and Western Esotericism* (New York: Continuum, 2005), 199.

36. Menuhin letter to the International Arts League of South Africa, Sept. 25, 1957, Foyle Menuhin Archive.

37. Menuhin letter to the International Arts League of South Africa, copy sent to Iyengar followed by a "Message from Yehudi Menuhin," introducing Iyengar and yoga to an audience, n.d., RIMYI Archive.

38. Menuhin letter to Iyengar, Jan. 4, 1960, RIMYI Archive.

39. Menuhin letter to Iyengar, Jan. 4. Menuhin must have been referring to Geeta Iyengar (1944–2018), who indeed later became a great yoga teacher and the codirector of RIMYI with her brother Prashant.

40. Iyengar letter to Menuhin, July 15, 1960, Foyle Menuhin Archive.

41. Iyengar letter to Menuhin, July 15.

42. Iyengar letter to Menuhin, July 23, 1960, Foyle Menuhin Archive.

43. Iyengar letter to Menuhin, July 23.

44. This marriage ended in divorce. Zamira stayed happily married to her second husband, Jonathan Benthall. As of this writing, she still lives in London.

45. Menuhin letter to Iyengar, Jan. 7, 1961, RIMYI Archive.

46. Menuhin letter to Iyengar, Jan. 7.

47. Menuhin letter to Iyengar, Apr. 18, 1961, RIMYI Archive.

48. Menuhin letter to Iyengar, Apr. 18.

49. Menuhin letter to Iyengar, Apr. 18.

50. Menuhin letter to Iyengar, Dec. 23, 1962, RIMYI Archive.

51. The typescript of the complete transcript is in the Foyle Menuhin Archive.

52. "Interview with Sri Prashant Iyengar on Yehudi Menuhin," *Yoga Rahasya* 23/2 (2016): 32.

53. Kofi Busia, "B. K. S. Iyengar Biography," *Kofi Busia* (website), accessed July 5, 2018, http://www.kofibusia.com/iyengarbiography/iyengarbio14.php.

54. Letter from Menuhin to Mr. Lobo of RIMYI, Sept. 30, 1974, RIMYI Archive.

55. Menuhin's personal message for the inauguration of RIMYI on Nov. 22, 1974, Foyle Menuhin Archive.

56. B. K. S. Iyengar, *Light on Pranayama: The Yogic Art of Breathing* (New York: Crossroad Publishing, 2001), xiii.

57. B. K. S. Iyengar, *Light on the Yoga Sutras* (London: Thorsons, 1996), vii.

58. Menuhin letter to Iyengar, Sept. 16, 1965, RIMYI Archive.

59. Menuhin letter to Iyengar, Dec. 28, 1966, RIMYI Archive.

60. Menuhin letter to Iyengar, Dec. 28. Menuhin must have been referring to the aftermath of the 1965 Indo-Pakistani war.

61. Menuhin letter to Iyengar, Apr. 1, 1968, with attached letter to Prime Minister Indira Gandhi, RIMYI Archive.

62. Menuhin letter to Iyengar, Apr. 1.

63. Menuhin, *Unfinished Journey*, 273.

64. Menuhin's text for the inauguration of RIMYI regarding yoga and music, Nov. 22, 1974, RIMYI Archive.

65. Menuhin BBC interview with Aley Hasan on Indian music, Nov. 17, 1960, Foyle Menuhin Archive.

66. Burton, *Menuhin*, 328.

67. Menuhin's message in Ravi Shankar's "Homage to Alaudin Khan" program, Dec. 3, 1972, Foyle Menuhin Archive.

68. Introduction to Shankar's 1968 [auto?] biography, quoted in Rolf P. Steiger and Hans-Ulrich Tschanz, *Gstaad and the Menuhins* (Wabern-Bern: Benteli Verlags AG, 2006), 136.

69. Yehudi Menuhin, "The Reification of Rhythm," review of *Indian Music and the West*, by Gerry Farrell, *Times Higher Education Supplement*, July 11, 1997, Foyle Menuhin Archive.

70. Menuhin letter to Shankar, Jan. 1998, Foyle Menuhin Archive.

71. Menuhin letter to Iyengar, Mar. 30, 1998, Foyle Menuhin Archive.

72. Produced by the Ford Foundation, the live show *Omnibus* from New York City is probably best remembered today for such celebrated hosts as Leonard Bernstein and Alastair Cooke.

73. Menuhin, *Unfinished Journey*, 360. A raga forms the melodic framework for improvisation in classical Indian music.

74. Menuhin, 360.

75. Menuhin, *Fiddler's Moll*, 218–19.

76. Burton, *Menuhin*, 330.

77. Burton, 385–86.

78. Newcombe, *Yoga in Britain*, 139. For more information on the important cultural connections between Menuhin's influence in promoting Shankar and the wider impact of Indian music, spirituality, and yoga on George Harrison and other popular music figures of the 1960s and 1970s, see Newcombe's entire chapter 5, "Yoga in Popular Music and the 'Counter-Culture' (the 1960s and '70s)," 134–76.

79. Menuhin, *Unfinished Journey*, 275

80. Menuhin, 274. The actual title of this work by Jacob Gade is "Tango Jalousie." Menuhin doesn't indicate the year of this BBC broadcast.

81. Menuhin, 274.

82. Menuhin, 274.

83. Menuhin, 427.

84. Menuhin left a recorded legacy to document his musical travels into Indian music and jazz, including around seventy-five pieces with Shankar and Grappelli, along with other jazz musicians like Duke Ellington, Oscar Peterson, and Johnny Dankworth. See Bruno Monsaingeon, *Passion Menuhin: The Album of a Life*, 247. Berlin: EuroArts Music International, 2016. Published with *The Menuhin Century*. Warner Classics 0825646777068, 2016.

85. Yehudi Menuhin, Festival of India message, 1985, Foyle Menuhin Archive.

Notes to Chapter 4

1. Such as *The Music of Man* (1979), *Menuhin Music Guides* (1980s), and *The Violin* (1996). His important essays and lectures from 1949 to 1970 have been collected in *Theme and Variations* (1972). See the bibliography for a list of Menuhin's books.

2. Yehudi Menuhin, *Violin: Six Lessons with Yehudi Menuhin* (London: Faber and Faber, 1971), 15.

3. Yehudi Menuhin, *Unfinished Journey: Twenty Years Later* (New York: Fromm International Publishing, 1997), 34.

4. Yehudi Menuhin, "Be Sensitive to Small Sensations," *Music Insider Newsletter*, Mar. 1982, Foyle Menuhin Archive, Royal Academy of Music, London.

5. B. K. S. Iyengar, *Light on the Yoga Sutras of Patañjali* (London: Thorsons, 1996), 159.

6. Menuhin, *Unfinished Journey*, 376.

7. Humphrey Burton, *Menuhin: A Life* (London: Faber and Faber, 2000), 411.

8. Menuhin, *Unfinished Journey*, 385.

9. Menuhin, 383.

10. Menuhin, 375.

11. Menuhin, 373.

12. Menuhin, 374–75.

13. Menuhin, 375.

14. Menuhin, 375.

15. Menuhin, 379.

16. Menuhin, 379.

17. Menuhin, 380.

18. Burton, *Menuhin*, 415.

19. Burton, 388.

20. Burton, 389.

21. Yehudi Menuhin School Student Interview Transcripts, 1964, Foyle Menuhin Archive.

22. Menuhin quote in Irving Kolodin, "Education on the Menuhin Plan," Nov. 27, 1965, Foyle Menuhin Archive.

23. Yehudi Menuhin, "Man: By Definition a Religious Animal: Of the Sacredness of Consciousness, Conscience and Choice," *World Faiths Insight* (Spring 1981): 3, Foyle Menuhin Archive.

24. Menuhin, *Unfinished Journey*, 425.

25. Natasha Boyarsky, violin instructor, Yehudi Menuhin School, unpublished interview with Catherine MacGregor and Kristin Wendland, Surrey, England, Mar. 15, 2018.

26. "Remembering Yehudi," Yehudi Menuhin School Archive, Aug. 10, 2016, https://www.yehudimenuhinschool.co.uk.

27. Menuhin, quoted in Burton, *Menuhin*, 465.

28. Lysy had already started other chamber groups in Argentina, including the Camerata Bariloche in 1967 and Camerata Lysy in 1971.

29. Lisa Yancich, unpublished interview with Catherine MacGregor, Atlanta, GA, Oct. 2017; and email communication with the author, Aug. 18–20, 2019.

30. Christopher Pulgram unpublished interview with Catherine MacGregor, Atlanta, GA, Dec. 2017; and email communication with the author, Aug. 18–20, 2019.

31. Menuhin, *Violin*, 11.

32. Menuhin, 14.

33. Menuhin, 14.

34. Menuhin, 15.

35. Menuhin, 16.

36. Menuhin, 17.

37. Iyengar explains and demonstrates two approaches to this technique, *surya bhedana pranayama* (breath inhaled through the right "sun" channel of the nose) and *nadi sodhana pranayama* (alternate breathing through the right and left nostrils while partially blocking the aperture with the thumb tip) in *Light on Yoga*, rev. ed. (New York: Schocken Books, 1979), 443–48.

38. Menuhin, *Violin*, 17.

39. Menuhin, 18. Author's note: A violinist must constantly and subtly shift the position of their fingers on the strings in order to play with perfect intonation, which requires concentrated listening and complete physical presence in the moment.

40. Menuhin, Yehudi Menuhin Violin Tutorial, "Lesson Six," YouTube video, accessed July 7, 2020, https://www.youtube.com/watch?v=O7BZV1btlK4&list=PLDLWkEm-ud7RedkBpuYEHasFuueIVGJdx.

41. Menuhin, *Violin*, 126.

42. Menuhin, 139.

43. In the digital version of this book, I illustrate the following discussion of Menuhin's yoga-centered approach in *Life Class* with videos enacting his instructions for some of the exercises. Catherine MacGregor performs in the videos while I narrate Menuhin's instructions. MacGregor's commentary and interpretation of the exercises are included below the video links. I am grateful for the help, expertise, and support from staff at the Emory Center for Digital Scholarship in producing these videos.

44. Yehudi Menuhin, *Life Class* (London: Heinemann, 1986), ix.

45. Menuhin, 6.

46. Menuhin, 27–30.

47. Menuhin, 34–35.

48. Menuhin, 96.

49. Menuhin, 96.

50. Menuhin, 99.

51. Menuhin, 109.

52. Menuhin, 108.

53. Menuhin, 123.

54. Menuhin, 124.

55. Iyengar, *Light on the Yoga Sutras of Patañjali*, 64.

56. Menuhin, *Life Class*, 124–25.

57. Iyengar, *Light on the Yoga Sutras of Patañjali*, 159.

58. Menuhin, *Life Class*, 125.

59. Iyengar, *Light on the Yoga Sutras of Patañjali*, 179.

60. Menuhin, *Life Class*, 126.

61. Menuhin, 127.

62. Menuhin, 129.

63. Menuhin, 131.

64. Menuhin, 135.

65. Menuhin, 136–37.

66. Patañjali's yoga sutra 1.20 cites *shraddha* (trust, faith) as the first of the five yoga virtues, followed by *virya* (vigor, strength), *smrti* (memory, recollection), *samadhi* (profound meditation, perfect absorption), and *prajna* (awareness of real knowledge). Iyengar, *Light on the Yoga Sutras of Patañjali*, 73–74.

67. Menuhin, *Life Class*, 137.

68. Menuhin, 139–41.

69. Menuhin, 141.

70. Menuhin, 143.

71. Menuhin, 145.

72. Menuhin, 145–46.

73. Menuhin, 147.

74. Menuhin, 148.

75. Menuhin, 148.

76. BBC interview with Aley Hasan, Nov. 17, 1960, Foyle Menuhin Archive.

77. Such as Yehudi Menuhin, "Indian and Western Music: An Attempt to Forecast Future Trends," *Hemisphere: An Asian-Australian Magazine*, Sydney, Australia, Apr. 1962: 2–7. Foyle Menuhin Archive.

78. "Mr. Menuhin's Notes for Sleeve of Record with Ravi Shankar," July 5, 1966, typescript, Foyle Menuhin Archive.

79. Yehudi Menuhin, "An Ancient Art and a New Experience," Ravi Shankar's program in honor of Allauddin Khan, Dec. 3, 1972, Foyle Menuhin Archive.

80. While Menuhin dates these East-West common origins to around one thousand years ago, archeologists have indeed traced migration of near-eastern farmers into southeastern Europe about eight thousand years ago, where the two cultures mixed in the area of the Danube, and "Southeastern Europe continued to be a nexus between east and west after the arrival of farmers." Iain Mathieson et al., "The Genomic History of Southeastern Europe," *Nature* 555 (2018): 197–203, https://www.nature.com/articles/nature25778.

81. Interestingly and coincidentally, both Menuhin and Shankar encountered Enesco's sphere of influence in the early 1930s in Paris, as Enesco used to listen to Shankar rehearsing Indian music and Enesco took Menuhin to the Colonial Exhibition in Paris in 1932 to hear the Indonesian Gamelan Orchestra.

82. Menuhin, "Mr. Menuhin's Notes for Sleeve of Record with Ravi Shankar," Foyle Menuhin Archive.

83. Menuhin letter to Ravi Shankar, Oct. 14, 1994, Foyle Menuhin Archive.

84. Menuhin letter to Ravi Shankar, Oct. 14.

85. Burton, *Menuhin*, 479.

86. Yehudi Menuhin, "The Reification of Rhythm," review of *Indian Music and the West*, by Gerry Farrell, *Times Higher Education Supplement*, July 11, 1997, Foyle Menuhin Archive.

87. Menuhin, "Indian and Western Music," Foyle Menuhin Archive.

88. Menuhin, "Indian and Western Music."

89. Menuhin, "Indian and Western Music."

90. Yehudi Menuhin, typescript of Ford Foundation *Omnibus* program, Salt Lake City, Mar. 16, 1955, Foyle Menuhin Archive.

91. Yehudi Menuhin, "The Music of India," in *Theme and Variations* (New York: Stein and Day, 1972), 76.

92. Yehudi Menuhin, "The Music of India, an Ancient Art Form," *New York Times*, Apr. 17, 1955; and "Indian and Western Music," Foyle Menuhin Archive.

93. Menuhin letter to Dr. Satyanath in response to the BBC World Phone-In Program, Nov. 4, 1983, Foyle Menuhin Archive.

94. Menuhin letter to Dr. Satyanath. Menuhin is making a veiled reference here to the equal temperament tuning of the modern piano, which results in all the intervals sounding slightly out of tune compared to the mathematically pure intervals of the Indian tuning system of just intonation.

95. Menuhin, "The Music of India, an Ancient Art Form."

96. Yehudi Menuhin, 1985 Festival of India message, undated typescript message, Foyle Menuhin Archive.

97. Menuhin, 1985 Festival of India message.

Notes to Chapter 5

1. B. K. S. Iyengar, *Light on Yoga*, rev. ed. (New York: Schocken Books, 1979), 31.

2. Yehudi Menuhin, *Unfinished Journey: Twenty Years Later* (New York: Fromm International Publishing, 1997), 414.

3. Yehudi Menuhin, quoted on the Live Music Now website, accessed June 29, 2020, http://www.livemusicnow.org.uk/live-music-now. See also the archival video of Menuhin performing for the Allied troops embedded on the LMN homepage.

4. Menuhin, *Unfinished Journey*, 420–21.

5. Humphrey Burton, *Menuhin: A Life* (London: Faber and Faber, 2000), 476.

6. Today the program has spread to eleven countries, and its current mission has broadened Menuhin's inclusive approach to align with the concepts of music education developed by the Hungarian composer, ethnomusicologist, and teacher Zoltán Kodály (1882–1967). See http://www.menuhin-foundation.com/mus-e/.

7. Menuhin Foundation Mission Statement, accessed Aug. 25, 2019, http://www.menuhin-foundation.com/.

8. Menuhin, quoted in Burton, *Menuhin*, 476.

9. Burton, *Menuhin*, 360.

10. "Musical Living, Nine Words: Yehudi Menuhin's Definitions," *Music Insider*, n.d., but the clipping must be from 1971 since the reporter cites Menuhin's speech to the IMC in Moscow. Foyle Menuhin Archive, Royal Academy of Music, London.

11. Menuhin, *Unfinished Journey*, 306.

12. Menuhin, 455.

13. Menuhin, 455.

14. Menuhin, 456.

15. Menuhin, 454.

16. Menuhin, 454.

17. Menuhin, 453.

18. Yehudi Menuhin, "Creative Attitude," speech at the US Embassy in Paris, Jan. 3, 1969, Foyle Menuhin Archive.

19. Yehudi Menuhin, "Heaven on Earth," presidential address to the Conservation Society, Royal Commonwealth Hall, Nov. 1, 1969, Foyle Menuhin Archive. A version of this speech with same title was published in the collection of Menuhin's important essays and lectures from 1949 to 1970 titled *Theme and Variations* (New York: Stein and Day, 1972), 135–46.

20. "Yehudi Menuhin, Journeys with a Violin," Royal Academy of Music Centenary, video, 2016.

21. I am grateful to Herr Rolf Steiger, director of the Menuhin Center Saanen, for walking me through this journey with Menuhin on Jan. 3, 2020, and for enlightening me on so many facets of Menuhin's life in the Saanenland.

22. Menuhin, *Unfinished Journey*, 264.

23. Yehudi Menuhin, "University of Madras Message In Celebration of the 81st Birthday of His Holiness Sri Chandrasekarendra Sarasvati," Nov. 1974, Foyle Menuhin Archive.

24. Menuhin, *Unfinished Journey*, 264.

25. "Biography," *Constantin Bruner* (website), accessed Aug. 24, 2019, https://www.constantinbrunner.net/en/biography/.

26. Yehudi Menuhin, "King's College: Music and Religion," notes, 1991, Foyle Menuhin Archive.

27. Menuhin letter to Dr. Drury, King's College, Feb. 1, 1991, Foyle Menuhin Archive.

28. Theosophical Society in America, website, accessed Aug. 24, 2019, https://www.theosophical.org/. Notably, the international headquarters of the Theosophical Society is in Chennai, India, and it published Rohit Mehta's translation and commentary of the Patañjali yoga sutras cited in the bibliography.

29. The Foyle Menuhin Archive at the Royal Academy of Music in London holds many such documents, most of which are catalogued and organized in boxes and folders, such as "Speeches and Addresses 1951–1969," but some are still uncatalogued, such as the box titled "Philosophy and Religion."

30. Yehudi Menuhin, luncheon address to the World Movement for World Federal Government, Sydney, Australia, June 4, 1951, Foyle Menuhin Archive.

31. Yehudi Menuhin, "Art and Science as Related Concepts," lecture, Jan. 30, 1959, Royal Institution of Great Britain, Foyle Menuhin Archive. A version of this talk with same title was published in *Theme and Variations*, 110–32.

32. Yehudi Menuhin, "Is an Unspiritual Education Possible?" Irvine Memorial Lecture, St. Andrews University, Oct. 25, 1967, Foyle Menuhin Archive.

33. Yehudi Menuhin, "How Does the Creative Artist Express the Spirit of His Time," address at the Dean of Windsor's Symposium June 4–7, 1973, Foyle Menuhin Archive.

34. Yehudi Menuhin, "Creativity," lecture, Smithsonian Resident Associate Program, Apr. 26, 1974, Foyle Menuhin Archive.

35. Menuhin, "Creativity."

36. Yehudi Menuhin, "A Recognition of Art as Hope," Gillies lecture, Lecture Hall of the Royal Scottish Museum in Edinburgh, July 20, 1982, Foyle Menuhin Archive.

37. Yehudi Menuhin, "Message to the Conference on Music, Mathematics, and Mysticism," sponsored by the Wrekin Trust, Hereford, UK, Mar. 1985, Foyle Menuhin Archive.

38. Yehudi Menuhin, "Tolerance," Adam lecture, King's College London, Feb. 26, 1987, Foyle Menuhin Archive.

39. Yehudi Menuhin, "Man: By Definition a Religious Animal: Of the Sacredness of Consciousness, Conscience and Choice," first delivered as the Francis Younghusband memorial lecture to the World Congress of Faiths at Westminster Abbey, July 18, 1980, and then printed in *World Faiths Insight* (Spring 1981): 3–11, Foyle Menuhin Archive.

40. Yehudi Menuhin, "On Oneness," typescript; "Escape the Fate of the Dinosaur," *The Times*, Aug. 21, 1989; and "Pray for an Orphaned Race," *The Times*, Aug. 22, 1989, Foyle Menuhin Archive. The complete essay was also translated to German as "Eins-sein" by Helmut Viebrick in Sept. 1989 for Goethe Universität, Frankfurt, and to French by Mdme. Madeline Santschi (n.d.).

41. Yehudi Menuhin, "Human Creativity," unpublished essay, 1993, Foyle Menuhin Archive.

42. Yehudi Menuhin, "Some Ephemeral Thoughts on Tolerance and Peace For Madame Lalumiere," 1994, Foyle Menuhin Archive.

43. "Guruji on Iyengar Yoga: Edited Transcript of Guruji's Address on his 70th Birthday in 1978" [*sic*, the year was 1988], *Yoga Rahasya* 27/1 (2020): 22.

44. Menuhin, "Man: By Definition a Religious Animal."

45. Menuhin letter to Clifford Longley, *The Times*, Aug. 15, 1989, Foyle Menuhin Archive.

46. Menuhin, "Escape the Fate of the Dinosaur."

47. Menuhin, "Escape the Fate of the Dinosaur."

48. Menuhin, "Pray for an Orphaned Race."

49. Menuhin, "Man: By Definition a Religious Animal."

50. Menuhin, "Man: By Definition a Religious Animal."

51. Menuhin, "Man: By Definition a Religious Animal."

52. "Guruji on Iyengar Yoga," *Yoga Rahasya* 27/1 (2020): 23.

53. Menuhin, "Man: By Definition a Religious Animal."

54. Menuhin, "Man: By Definition a Religious Animal."

55. Menuhin letter to Dr. Drury, King's College, Feb. 1, 1991.

56. Menuhin letter to Dr. Drury.

57. Yehudi Menuhin, "The Meaning of Life," fax to *Life* magazine, Aug. 20, 1991, Foyle Menuhin Archive. It's interesting to note this was the last "new"

communication technology Menuhin used. To my knowledge, he never made the leap to email and the Internet.

58. Menuhin, "The Meaning of Life."

59. Yehudi Menuhin, "The Meaning of Life," fax to Sichtermann International Publishing House, Oct. 16, 1991, Foyle Menuhin Archive.

60. Menuhin, "The Meaning of Life."

61. Yehudi Menuhin, handwritten answer on Paul Rifkin letter, n.d., Foyle Menuhin Archive.

62. Yehudi Menuhin, "Endless Time," unpublished paper, n.d., Foyle Menuhin Archive.

63. Menuhin letter to Iyengar, Apr. 1, 1968, outlining his BBC India project vision, Foyle Menuhin Archive.

64. Menuhin, "Endless Time."

65. Yehudi Menuhin, "Shanta Rao and the Dances of South India," script, presentation at MoMA, New York, Apr. 26, 1955, Foyle Menuhin Archive.

66. Yehudi Menuhin, "The Twain Shall Meet," *Saturday Review*, Jan. 31, 1953, Foyle Menuhin Archive.

67. Menuhin, "The Growing Interest of Western Nations in Indian Music Dance," *Manchurian Guardian*, Oct. 28, 1959, revised for the Asia Society of New York and reprinted in the *Indian Student* (1960), Foyle Menuhin Archive.

68. Menuhin, "Endless Time."

69. Yehudi Menuhin, "The Music of India, an Ancient Art Form," manuscript edited from his article in the *New York Times*, April 17, 1955, Foyle Menuhin Archive.

70. Yehudi Menuhin, "Mr. Menuhin's Notes for Sleeve of Record with Ravi Shankar," July 5, 1966, Foyle Menuhin Archive.

71. Yehudi Menuhin, "From East to West," *Times Supplement on the Arts in the Commonwealth*, Sept. 13, 1965, Foyle Menuhin Archive.

72. Menuhin, "Endless Time."

73. Yehudi Menuhin, "An Ancient Art and a New Experience," program notes for Ravi Shankar's Homage to Allauddin Khan concert, Dec. 3, 1972, Foyle Menuhin Archive.

74. Menuhin, "University of Madras Message In Celebration of the 81st Birthday of His Holiness Sri Chandrasekarendra Sarasvati."

75. Yehudi Menuhin, "My Prayer," four-page typescript, n.d., Foyle Menuhin Archive.

Notes to the Epilogue

1. Yehudi Menuhin, *Unfinished Journey: Twenty Years Later* (New York: Fromm International Publishing, 1997), 229.

2. Menuhin, 263.

3. Menuhin, 263.

4. Menuhin, 263.

5. Menuhin, 263.

6. Menuhin, 437.

7. "Intermission," *Intermission: Music, Movement, and Mindfulness*, accessed Sept. 26, 2019, https://www.intermissionsessions.com/.

8. Nicola Benedetti, violinist, interview with Catherine MacGregor and Kristin Wendland, London, UK, Mar. 16, 2018.

9. See "Nicola Benedetti/Recordings," *Nicola Benedetti* (website), accessed Sept. 7, 2022, https://www.nicolabenedetti.co.uk/recordings-details/wynton-marsalis-violin-concerto-amp-fiddle-dance-suite. Since this book went into production, Benedetti also brings fresh ideas and energy as the newly-appointed director of the Edinburgh International Festival beginning in 2023.

10. Daniel Hope interview with Kristin Wendland and Catherine MacGregor, Nov. 1, 2018, Emory University.

11. "Daniel Hope: The Violinist," *Daniel Hope* (website), accessed Sept. 25, 2019, https://www.danielhope.com/the-musical-activist/.

12. Kaddish is a Jewish hymn of praise to God and is often associated with the ritual of mourning.

13. Hope interview; and also on his website, accessed Sept. 25, 2019, https://www.danielhope.com/listento/my-tribute-to-yehudi-menuhin/.

14. Heidi Senungetuk, interview with the author, Atlanta, GA, Sept. 2, 2022.

15. Senungetuk, interview with Kristin Wendland.

16. Eleanor Hope, quoted in Humphrey Burton, *Menuhin: A Life* (London: Faber and Faber, 2000), 464.

17. *The Bhagavad Gita*, XVI.2, trans. Winthrop Sargeant (Albany: State University of New York Press, 1994), 611.

Bibliography

Benthall, Zamira [nee Menuhin]. Interview. *Yoga Rahasya*, 23/2 (2016): 37–38.

"B. K. S. Iyengar Yoga." *B. K. S. Iyengar Yoga* (website). Accessed July 3, 2019. http://bksiyengar.com/.

"B. K. S. Iyengar 1918–2014: Timeline of B. K. S. Iyengar's Life." *Iyengar Yoga* (website). Accessed Jan. 8, 2020. http://iyengaryoga.org.uk/timeline/.

Bryant, Edwin F. *The Yoga Sutras of Patañjali*. New York: North Point Press, 2009.

Bühnemann, Gudrun. "Naga, Siddha and Sage: Visions of Patañjali as an Authority on Yoga." In *Yoga in Transformation*, eds. Karl Baier, Philipp A. Maas, and Karin Preisendanz, 575–622. Vienna: Vienna University Press, 2018. https://www.vandenhoeck-ruprecht-verlage.com/themen-entdecken/theologie/religionswissenschaft/16133/yoga-in-transformation.

Burton, Humphrey. *Menuhin: A Life*. London: Faber and Faber, 2000.

Burton-Hill, Clemency. "Who's Yehudi? Yehudi Menuhin BBC Documentary." Posted by Arthur Grumiaux. 2016. YouTube video. https://www.youtube.com/watch?v=0h0GkOP7ZUs.

Busia, Kofi. "B. K. S. Iyengar Biography." *Kofi Busia* (website). Accessed July 3, 2018. http://www.kofibusia.com/iyengarbiography/iyengarbio14.php.

Carrera, Jaganath. *Inside the Yoga Sutras*. Yogaville, VA: Integral Yoga Publications, 2008.

Clennell, Jake, dir. *Iyengar: The Man, Yoga, and The Student's Journey*. 2018; Clennell Films. Documentary film. http://iyengarmovie.com/.

Daniels, Robin. *Conversations with Menuhin*. New York: St. Martin's Press, 1979.

De Michelis, Elizabeth. *A History of Modern Yoga: Patañjali and Western Esotericism*. New York: Continuum, 2005.

De Michelis, Elizabeth, Suzanne Newcomb, and Mark Singleton. "Modern Yoga Research." Accessed Jan. 8, 2020. http://www.modernyogaresearch.org/.

Dubal, David. *Conversations with Menuhin: A Celebration on His 75th Birthday*. London: Heinemann, 1991.

Goldberg, Elliott. *The Path of Modern Yoga: The History of an Embodied Spiritual Practice*. Rochester, VT: Inner Traditions, 2016.

Goldberg, Michelle. *The Goddess Pose: The Audacious Life of Indra Devi, the Woman Who Helped Bring Yoga to the West*. New York: Vintage Books, 2016.

"Interview with Sri Prashant Iyengar on Yehudi Menuhin." *Yoga Rahasya* 23/2 (2016): 33–38.

"Iyengar: A Yogi's Life." *Google Arts and Culture*. Accessed July 7, 2020. https://artsandculture.google.com/exhibit/ZgLCKGRRbVhaJg.

Iyengar, B. K. S. *Astadala Yogamala, Collected Works*. Vol. 1, Articles, Lectures, Messages. New Delhi, India: Allied Publishers Private, 2000.

———. "CNN Interview with B. K. S. Iyengar." By Anjali Rao. *CNN Talk Asia*. June 3, 2012. YouTube video. https://www.youtube.com/watch?v=cXJEzPGZqo8.

———. "Guruji on Iyengar Yoga, Edited Transcript of Guruji's Address on His 70th Birthday in 1978" [*sic*, the year was 1988]. *Yoga Rahasya* 27/1 (2020): 22–33.

———. "The Historic Meeting." *Yoga Rahasya* 23/2 (2016): 9–17.

———. *Light on Life: The Yoga Journey to Wholeness, Inner Peace, and Ultimate Freedom*. [Emmaus, PA]: Rodale Books, 2005.

———. "Light on the Life of a Master." Interview with Harsh Desai. *The Tribune* (India). Dec. 4, 2005. http://www.tribuneindia.com/2005/20051204/spectrum/main1.htm.

———. *Light on Pranayama: The Yogic Art of Breathing*. New York: Crossroad Publishing, 2001.

———. *Light on Yoga*. Rev. ed. New York: Schocken Books, 1979.

———. *Light on the Yoga Sutras*. London: Thorsons, 1996.

———. *The Tree of Life*. Edited by Daniel Rivers-Moore. Boston: Shambala, 2002.

———. "You Have Taught Me How to Play the Violin." Interview with Rujuta Diwekar. Aug. 20, 2014. http://bangaloremirror.indiatimes.com/news/india/You-have-taught-me-how-to-play-the-violin/articleshow/40525332.cms.

Krishnamacharya, Tirumalai. *Yoga Makiranda*. Translated and edited by T. V. K. Desikachar. Chennai, India: MediaGaruda, 2011.

Magidoff, Robert. *Yehudi Menuhin*. 2nd ed. London: Robert Hale, 1973.

Mehta, Rohit. *Yoga: The Art of Integration; A Commentary on the Yoga Sutras of Patañjali*. Chennai, India: Theosophical Publishing House, 2011.

Menuhin, Diana. *Fiddler's Moll*. New York: St. Martin's Press, 1984.

Menuhin, Yehudi. *Life Class: Thoughts, Exercises, Reflections of an Itinerant Violinist*. London: Heinemann, 1986. Also published as *The Compleat Violinist*. New York: Summit Books, 1986.

———. *The Music of Man*. Sydney, Australia: Methuen, 1979.

———. *Theme and Variations*. New York: Stein and Day, 1972.

———. *Unfinished Journey: Twenty Years Later*. New York: Fromm International Publishing, 1997.

———. *The Violin*. Paris: Flammarion, 1996.

———. *Violin: Six Lessons with Yehudi Menuhin*. London: Faber and Faber, 1971.

Menuhin, Yehudi, and William Primrose. *Yehudi Menuhin Music Guides: The Violin and Viola*. New York: Schirmer Books, 1976.

Mohan, A. G. *Krishnamacharya: His Life and Teachings*. Boston: Shambala, 2010.

Mohan, A. G., with Ganesh Mohan, trans. *Yoga Yajnavalkya*. Svastha Yoga, 2013.

Monsaingeon, Bruno. *Passion Menuhin: The Album of a Life*. Berlin: EuroArts Music International, 2016. This multilingual work in German, French, and English was published in conjunction with the release of *The Menuhin Century*, Warner Classics 0825646777068, 2016.

————, dir. *Yehudi Menuhin: The Violin of the Century*. 1994; documentary film. Written by Bruno Monsaingeon. France: Ideale Audience.

Newcombe, Suzanne. "The Development of Modern Yoga: A Survey of the Field." *Religion Compass* 3/6 (2009): 986–1002. http://modernyogaresearch.org/wp-content/uploads/2016/05/Pre-Pub-Religion-Compass.pdf.

————. "The Revival of Yoga in Contemporary India." *Oxford Research Encyclopedias*. Accessed May 2017. https://oxfordre.com/religion/view/10.1093/acrefore/9780199340378.001.0001/acrefore-9780199340378-e-253.

————. "Spaces of Yoga: Towards a Non-Essentialist Understanding of Yoga." In *Yoga in Transformation: Historical and Contemporary Perspectives*, eds. Karl Baier, Philipp A. Maas, and Karin Preisendanz, 551–73. Göttingen: V&R unipress, Vienna University Press, 2018. https://www.vandenhoeck-ruprecht-verlage.com/themen-entdecken/theologie/religionswissenschaft/16133/yoga-in-transformation.

————. *Yoga in Britain: Stretching Spirituality and Educating Yogis*. Sheffield, UK: Equinox Publishing, 2019.

Palmer, Tony. *Menuhin: A Family Portrait*. London: Faber and Faber, 1991.

Rolfe, Lionel Menuhin. *The Menuhins: A Family Odyssey*. San Francisco: Panjandrum/Aris Books, 1978.

Sarbacker, Stuart Ray. *Tracing the Path of Yoga*. Albany: State University of New York Press, 2021.

Sargeant, Winthrop, trans. *The Bhagavad Gita*. Albany: State University of New York Press, 1994.

Singleton, Mark, and Ellen Goldberg, eds. *Gurus of Modern Yoga*. New York: Oxford University Press, 2014.

Singleton, Mark, and Jean Bryne, eds. *Yoga in the Modern World: Contemporary Perspectives*. London: Routledge, 2008.

Steiger, Rolf P., and Hans-Ulrich Tschanz. *Gstaad and the Menuhins*. Wabern-Bern: Benteli Verlags AG, 2006.

Swami Swatmarama. *Hatha Yoga Pradipika*. Translated by Pancham Sinh. Forgotten Books, 2008. Reprinted from the 1914 publication.

White, David Gordon. *The Yoga Sutra of Patañjali: A Biography*. Princeton, NJ: Princeton University Press, 2014.

"Yehudi Menuhin and B. K. S. Iyengar's Transformative Friendship." *Iyengar Yoga London* (blog). Accessed July 7, 2020. https://iymv.org/yehudi-menuhin-and-bks-iyengars-transformative-friendship/.

"Yehudi Menuhin: Journeys with a Violin." Documentary film for the Menuhin centennial celebration. London: Royal Academy of Music, 2016.

"Yehudi Menuhin." *Yehudi Menuhin* (website). Accessed July 7, 2020. https://www.menuhin.org/.

"Yehudi Menuhin: Six Violin Lessons." Posted by Richard Downs Jr. Updated Mar. 1, 2013. YouTube video. https://www.youtube.com/playlist?list=PLDLWk Em-ud7RedkBpuYEHasFuueIVGJdx.

Index